AF669861

Cell Therapy for Perinatal Brain Injury

Haruo Shintaku • Akira Oka • Makoto Nabetani
Editors

Cell Therapy for Perinatal Brain Injury

Springer

Editors
Haruo Shintaku
Department of Pediatrics
Osaka City University Graduate School of Medicine
Osaka, Japan

Akira Oka
Department of Pediatrics
University of Tokyo
Tokyo, Japan

Makoto Nabetani
Department of Pediatrics
Yodogawa Christian Hospital
Osaka, Japan

ISBN 978-981-10-1411-6 ISBN 978-981-10-1412-3 (eBook)
https://doi.org/10.1007/978-981-10-1412-3

Library of Congress Control Number: 2018930911

© Springer Nature Singapore Pte Ltd. 2018
This work is subject to copyright. All rights are reserved by the Publisher, whether the whole or part of the material is concerned, specifically the rights of translation, reprinting, reuse of illustrations, recitation, broadcasting, reproduction on microfilms or in any other physical way, and transmission or information storage and retrieval, electronic adaptation, computer software, or by similar or dissimilar methodology now known or hereafter developed.
The use of general descriptive names, registered names, trademarks, service marks, etc. in this publication does not imply, even in the absence of a specific statement, that such names are exempt from the relevant protective laws and regulations and therefore free for general use.
The publisher, the authors and the editors are safe to assume that the advice and information in this book are believed to be true and accurate at the date of publication. Neither the publisher nor the authors or the editors give a warranty, express or implied, with respect to the material contained herein or for any errors or omissions that may have been made. The publisher remains neutral with regard to jurisdictional claims in published maps and institutional affiliations.

Printed on acid-free paper

This Springer imprint is published by Springer Nature
The registered company is Springer Nature Singapore Pte Ltd.
The registered company address is: 152 Beach Road, #21-01/04 Gateway East, Singapore 189721, Singapore

Preface

Perinatal brain injury is a leading cause of cerebral palsy (CP), often resulting in lifelong disabilities. Because more than 90% of CP patients today survive into adulthood, the economic and social burdens associated with support for the patients and their families are significant, and therefore pathophysiological understanding of the disease and development of effective therapies are urgent public health needs. Perinatal hypoxic–ischemic encephalopathy (HIE) is an important cause of brain injury resulting from reduced cerebral blood flow at birth that leads to hypoxia and hypoglycemia in brain cells. Impaired uptake of glutamate by brain neurons results in intracellular calcium accumulation, which ultimately causes irreversible damage. To date, hypothermia therapy has been the only effective treatment for HIE to prevent the development of CP. A recent publication in the United States [1], however, indicated benefits of autologous umbilical cord blood stem cell transplantation combined with hypothermia therapy for HIE, drawing attention to cell therapy for perinatal brain injury. This book, coauthored by leading physicians in the field, is intended to provide comprehensive and concise information to readers on the most recent advances in cell therapy for perinatal brain injury, from basic stem cell biology to clinical essentials.

Stem cells in umbilical cord blood were first discovered by Japanese researchers, Nakahata and Ogawa, in [2]. This led to a report by Gluckman et al. in [3] on the first clinical success of cord blood transplantation (CBT) in a patient with Fanconi's anemia. Since then, various public and private cord blood banks have been established and have provided cord blood units for transplantation to more than 30,000 pediatric and adult patients. CBT quickly gained importance also in Japan after the foundation of the Japanese Cord Blood Bank Network in 1999. Although initially limited to hematological disorders, CBT has found its application in inherited metabolic disorders since the turn of this century. In 2005, Escolar et al. reported a significant survival benefit of CBT in patients with early-stage infantile Krabbe disease [4]. According to their report, the 6-year mortality rate was 0% in 11 patients who underwent CBT from unrelated donors before the development of symptoms as opposed to an untreated cohort of 190 children who all died before reaching 8 years of age. In 2008, the potential of cord blood stem cells to differentiate into neural cells was reported [5] and offered promising new uses of CBT and bone marrow transplantation in inherited metabolic diseases as reviewed by Prasad and Kurtzberg in [6]. Along with the reported clinical successes in inherited metabolic diseases, researchers in the field of brain injury began to devote their efforts to scientific studies on the role of CBT in central nervous system injuries associated with hypoxia and ischemia, exploring the potential of cord blood stem cells for brain regeneration.

In vitro experiments in [7] and [8] demonstrated the expression of neural and normal cell markers in human nucleated cord blood cells and the expression of oligodendroglial and astrocytic features in $CD34^+$ and other cord blood stem cells. Through in vivo studies using a rat model of ischemic stroke, an improved outcome after intravenous administration of human cord blood stem cells to male rats was demonstrated in [9], and reduction in spastic paresis after intraperitoneal transplantation of human cord blood stem cells within 24 h of injury was reported in [10]. Although incorporation of the transplanted human mononuclear cells primarily around the lesioned brain area and engraftment 14 days posttransplantation were demonstrated, significant changes in lesion volume or differentiation into astrocytes were not observed. Thus, differentiation of human nucleated cord blood cells into neural cells observed in vitro was not confirmed in in vivo studies. These laboratory results are consistent with clinical data in humans. Kurtzberg et al. reported in [11] that donor-derived cells had differentiated into vessels, microglia, and choroid plexus cells but not into neuroectodermal cells (i.e., neurons, astrocytes, and oligodendrocytes) in the brain of a female infant with Krabbe disease who received CBT. These studies collectively suggest that transplanted cells do cross the blood–brain barrier and engraft in the brain but do not restore the lost function by differentiating into neural cells. Rather, it seems that these cells achieve clinical benefits through some other mechanisms that facilitate the repair of surrounding tissues.

The clinical efficacy of CBT in CP patients has recently been demonstrated. Autologous CBT in 20 CP patients in a study by Lee et al. in [12] and allogeneic CBT in 31 CP patients in a study by Min et al. in [13] both led to neurological improvements without serious adverse events. In the most recent study published in 2014, Cotten et al. [1] isolated stem cells from the autologous cord blood and administered them to cooled infants with moderate or severe HIE. The treatment was safe and resulted in significantly better intact survival with Bayley III scores of ≥85 compared with infants who received hypothermia therapy alone, although overall survival was not significantly different between the two groups. So, how does CBT work in the treatment of CP? Regulation of microglial response and facilitation of axonal sprouting have been indicated by recent studies. These findings suggest that the cord blood is capable of repairing brain damage through multiple endogenous pathways.

Although much of today's laboratory research focuses on embryonic stem cells and induced pluripotent stem cells that can differentiate into any type of tissue, these approaches have limitations in terms of clinical application to the treatment of perinatal HIE because they require a longer preparation and culture time, which may not fit within the short time window for optimal therapy. Allogeneic cells may be stocked in advance, but this approach always comes with the risk of immune rejection. In contrast, cord blood, once considered medical waste, is an ideal source of stem cells for perinatal HIE as it obviates the ethical issues associated with the use of fetal cells and at the same time reduces the risk of rejection if autologous cord blood is used.

On August 6, 2014, the first clinical trial protocol for autologous cord blood stem cell therapy for neonatal HIE was approved in Japan. This trial is a new multicenter effort involving 11 CP research groups across Japan collaborating at all levels from the nonclinical to clinical phases to evaluate the safety and efficacy of autologous cord blood stem cell transplantation in HIE infants in combination with hypothermia therapy. Perinatal HIE is a leading cause of CP, and severe HIE occurs in one to six cases per 1000 live births. Despite effective treatment such as hypothermia therapy, severe sequelae still develop in 50% of patients. Because no effective treatment exists once brain damage has been established and CP symptoms have developed, neonatal management before the establishment of damage is crucial. In this context, CBT, in combination with hypothermia therapy, is a promising cell-based regenerative approach for preventing CP associated with perinatal brain injury.

References

1. Cotten CM. et al. Feasibility of autologous cord blood cells for infants with hypoxic-ischemic encephalopathy. J Pediatr. 2014;164(5):973–9.
2. Nakahata T, Ogawa M: Hemopoietic colony-forming cells in umbilical cord blood with extensive capability to generate mono- and multipotential hemopoietic progenitors. J Clin Invest. 1982; 70(6): 1324–8.
3. Gluckman E, et al. Hematopoietic Reconstitution in a Patient with Fanconi's Anemia by Means of Umbilical-Cord Blood from an HLA-Identical Sibling. NEJM. 1989; 321:1174–8.
4. Escolar et al. Transplantation of umbilical-cord blood in babies with infantile Krabbe's disease. NEJM 2005;352(20):2069–81.
5. Domanska-Januck K et al. A novel, neural potential of non-hematopoietic human umbilical cord blood stem cells. Int J Dev Biol 2008;52:237–48 (review)
6. Prasad V, Kurtzberg J.B Cord blood and bone marrow transplantation in inherited metabolic diseases: scientific basis, current status and future directions. Jnl Hematology 2009;148:356–72.
7. Sanchez-Ramos JR et al. Expression of neural markers in human umbilical cord blood. Exp Neurol. 2001;171:109–15.
8. Buzańska L et al. Human cord blood-derived cells attain neuronal and glial features in vitro. J Cell Sci. 2002;115:2131–8.
9. Chen J et al. Intravenous administration of human umbilical cord blood reduces behavioral deficits after stroke in rats. Stroke 2001;32:2682–8.
10. Meier C. et al. Spastic paresis after perinatal brain damage in rats is reduced by human cord blood mononuclear cells. Pediatr Res 2006;59:244–9.
11. Kurtzberg J, et al. Umbilical cord blood cells engraft and differentiate in neural tissues after human transplantation. Biology of Blood and Marrow Transplantation 2003;9:128–129.

12. Lee YH et al. Safety and feasibility of countering neurological impairment by intravenous administration of autologous cord blood in cerebral palsy. 2012 J Transl Med. 2012;23;10:58.
13. Min K et al. Umbilical cord blood therapy potentiated with erythropoietin for children with cerebral palsy: a double-blind, randomized, placebo-controlled trial. 2013 Stem Cells. 2013;31(3):581–91.

Osaka, Japan Haruo Shintaku, M.D., Ph.D.

Preface

With the advancement of prenatal obstetric care and postnatal intensive neonatal care, the incidence of cerebral palsy (CP) has been decreasing in developed countries. In fact, the incidence of CP in Okinawa Prefecture, which is in the southwestern part of Japan, was reported as 1.5 per 1000 live births between 2007 and 2009 [1], which corresponds to two thirds of the figure between 1995 and 2001. Because the progress of perinatal medicine covers wide-ranging aspects, it seems difficult to ascribe the improvement to any new specific technique. Accumulated evidence confirms the protective effects of hypothermia therapy on neonatal hypoxic–ischemic encephalopathy, and the therapy has been introduced as standard care in current clinical settings in Japan, reasonably contributing to the improved outcomes to a certain extent.

The Japan Obstetric Compensation System for Cerebral Palsy, which is a government-supported system, started registration of infants born after 2009 who suffered from CP possibly related to delivery. The registration reports approximately 1500 infants born between 2009 and 2011 who were diagnosed as having severe CP before the age of 5 years and fulfilling the conditions of the compensation by the system. This compensation system does not enroll infants born before 28 gestation weeks, and therefore caution is necessary when we interpret the figure. It is indisputable, however, that a significant number of infants still suffer from neonatal encephalopathy, requiring development of novel therapeutic approaches.

In this regard, we have remarked on the potential of stem cell therapy as early pioneers. After encouraging data in animal models reported by Dr. Tsuji [2], Dr. Shintaku organized a research group called the Neonatal Encephalopathy Consortium, Japan, consisting of neonatologists, neuroscientists, and pediatricians, and initiated a **feasibility** study using autologous umbilical cord blood stem cells. This special monograph is a product of the research group's work, reflecting their discussions and providing updated information on stem cell therapy applied to neonatal hypoxic–ischemic encephalopathy.

We truly appreciate the dedication of all contributors and congratulate their accomplishment as shown in this book.

References

1. The Japan Obstetric Compensation System for Cerebral Palsy Committee Report
2. Department of Regenerative Medicine and Tissue Engineering, National Cerebral and Cardiovascular Center

Tokyo, Japan Akira Oka, M.D., Ph.D.

Contents

Chapter 1
Clinical Trial of Autologous Cord Blood Cell Therapy for Neonatal Hypoxic Ischemic Encephalopathy (HIE)

Masahiro Tsuji and Haruo Shintaku

Abstract Cell-based therapy is attracting attention not only for its regenerative property but also for its long therapeutic time window. A growing number of studies in animal models with brain injuries have shown that cell therapies are beneficial. Among the variety of cell types to be used for cell therapies, autologous umbilical cord blood cells (UCBCs) are the most feasible; UCB contains several types of stem cells, the collection of the UCB is totally noninvasive and no ethical issues are involved, and UCBCs have no tumorigenicity. More than 20 preclinical studies have examined the effects of human UCBCs in models of neonatal brain injury; the majority of the studies were conducted in a rodent model of hypoxia-ischemia. Systemic administration of mononuclear fraction of UCB is the most extensively explored, and most of the studies have shown beneficial effects. Intravenous infusion of autologous non-cryopreserved volume- and red blood cell-reduced UCB is the most feasible method for cell therapy, especially when used at the acute phase of acute onset diseases. Fewer than ten clinical studies, including ours, using UCB for newborns with acute brain injury have been reported or listed on open registration websites, and only a few of the studies have reported the results, proving safety and feasibility and implying efficacy. No randomized control studies have been reported with respect to cell therapies during the newborn period. Further preclinical studies to optimize the treatment protocol and clinical trials to prove efficacy are warranted.

Keywords Clinical study · Cord blood cell · Cell infusion · Neonatal brain Injury

M. Tsuji, M.D., Ph.D. (✉)
Department of Regenerative Medicine and Tissue Engineering, National Cerebral and Cardiovascular Center, Suita, Osaka, Japan
e-mail: tsuji.masahiro.ri@ncvc.go.jp, mtsujimd@ybb.ne.jp

H. Shintaku, M.D., Ph.D.
Department of Pediatrics, Osaka City University Graduate School of Medicine, Abeno-ku, Osaka, Japan
e-mail: shintakuh@med.osaka-cu.ac.jp

© Springer Nature Singapore Pte Ltd. 2018

H. Shintaku et al. (eds.), *Cell Therapy for Perinatal Brain Injury*,
https://doi.org/10.1007/978-981-10-1412-3_1

1.1 Background of Cell Therapy for Neonatal Hypoxic-Ischemic Encephalopathy (HIE)

Acute brain injury may occur unexpectedly during the perinatal and neonatal periods. The conditions in which neonates present with acute brain dysfunction are collectively termed neonatal encephalopathy [1]. The signs and symptoms of brain dysfunction are recognized as an altered level of consciousness, weak muscle tone, impaired feeding, respiratory depression, and seizures. The vast majority of infants with neonatal encephalopathy are born with asphyxia, the causes of which are heterogeneous, such as low maternal blood pressure, premature placental abruption, compression of the umbilical cord, and severe congenital heart disease. The pathophysiology of neonatal encephalopathy is hypoxic-ischemic encephalopathy (HIE) in the majority of cases, up to 85% of neonatal encephalopathy cases, followed by neonatal stroke, which accounts for up to 10% of cases [2]. Children with severe neonatal HIE typically die or develop severe neurological sequelae such as cerebral palsy (CP), mental retardation, and epilepsy [3]. Children with moderate neonatal HIE suffer neurological sequelae in many cases; 81% have cognitive dysfunctions, and 30% have cerebral palsy when the survivors are assessed in their late teens [4].

Success in the translation of mild hypothermia was a landmark event for both neonatologists/pediatricians and neuroscientists. Before the introduction of mild hypothermia, treatment in neonatal intensive care units (NICUs) was merely supportive. Mild hypothermia was the first and is still the only treatment proven effective in large-scale randomized clinical trials [5, 6]. However, even if infants are treated with hypothermia, nearly half of them die or are left with moderate to severe neurological impairments. The therapeutic time window of hypothermia is within 6 h after birth. Therefore, there is an urgent need for the development of novel therapies for HIE. A review in year 2006 reported that nearly 700 therapies for acute stroke had proven effective in preclinical studies and that over 100 of them had been used in practice. Nevertheless, tissue plasminogen activator administered within 3 h after the onset of stroke was the only therapy proven effective in a clinical study [7]. Most of those therapies exert beneficial effects only when administered before the ischemic insult or immediately after the insult. Although some therapies demonstrate beneficial effects even when administered after certain periods of time, the therapeutic time window rarely exceed 6 h after the insult.

Cell-based therapy is attracting a lot of attention because not only of its regenerative property but also of the long therapeutic time window. Various studies in animal models with brain injuries have shown that cell therapies are beneficial. Those studies range from embryonic stem cells and induced pluripotent stem cells to mononuclear cell fractions of bone marrow and umbilical cord blood with respect to cell type, from culturing with several gene transfections and manipulations to simple separation of cells with gradient centrifugation with respect to cell preparation, from intracerebral transplantation to intravenous injection with respect to the administration route, and from xenotransplantation (from different species) to autologous transplantation (using one's own cells) with respect to the origin of cells.

In this chapter, after we briefly review the history of cell therapies in both preclinical and clinical studies, we review cell therapies using umbilical cord blood.

1.2 History of Cell Therapies for Brain Injury

1.2.1 Preclinical Studies on Cell Therapies for Neonatal Brain Injury

During the early days of research in stem cell therapy, most researchers conceived of the concept of "regeneration," in which transplanted stem cells proliferate and differentiate into new neurons and replace lost neurons. During the past decade, several other concepts have been added to the research, in which transplanted stem cells secrete a variety of trophic factors, suppress inflammation and modulate the immune response, and enhance endogenous neurogenesis and angiogenesis [8, 9]. A growing number of studies have demonstrated that the long-term survival of stem cells transplanted in the brain is not necessary [10–12]. Furthermore, many studies have shown that transition into the brain is not necessary in order that the administered cells exert beneficial effects on an injured brain [13, 14]. Currently conceived mechanisms of stem cell therapy are multimodal and not confined to regeneration. Hence the term "cell-based therapy" could be more appropriate than "regenerative therapy" at least in the field of acute brain injury.

More than 60 research articles on cell-based therapies for perinatal/neonatal brain injury have been published to date, and the number has been growing each year [15] (see Chap. 5 for details). The vast majority of those studies used rodent models of neonatal HIE. During the first decade since the first report in this field by [16], intracerebral transplantation of either the fetal brain tissue or neural stem cells (NSCs) was investigated. Systemic administration by intraperitoneal injection of cells was first reported by Meier et al. in [17]. Also, Meier et al. was the first to report the effects of umbilical cord blood (UCB) cells in neonatal models. Intravenous injection, a clinically feasible route of systemic administration, was first reported by Yasuhara et al. [18]. During the second decade, roughly equal numbers of studies using intracranial transplantation or systemic administration of stem cells have been reported in this research field. With respect to the donor cells, the mononuclear cell (MNC) fraction of human UCB and mesenchymal stem cells (MSCs) derived from rodent bone marrow (BM) have been most extensively investigated. MNCs are infused systematically and MSCs are transplanted intracranially in many of the studies.

Human UCB (hUCB) is the most extensively used cell source for preclinical research in neonatal brain injury. Over 20 studies have been reported in the literature [15, 19]. For details, refer to Chap. 5 in this textbook. Briefly, the majority of them have reported the beneficial effects of cell therapy in either morphological or behavioral evaluations or in both evaluations, although some reported no therapeutic effects. No adverse effects were noted. Two studies examined the effects of hUCB $CD34^+$ cells (hematopoietic/endothelial progenitor cells); three studies examined the effects of MSCs derived from hUCB; one study examined the effects of total nucleated cells; and all the other studies examined the effects of MNC fraction of hUCB. With respect to the administration route, cells were transplanted into brains in three studies with MSCs and two studies with MNCs; cells were injected systemically in other studies, intraperitoneally in approximately one third of the studies, and intravenously in approximately two thirds of the studies. The effective cell dose varied from 1.5×10^4 cells up to 1×10^8. Similarly, effective timing for the cell administration varied from 6 h to 7 days after the insult. Few studies have examined the optimal cell dose and timing of cell administration. Taking these findings together, among cell therapies for neonatal brain injury, systemic administration of hUCB MNCs is the most vigorously studied, and it has proven effective with no serious adverse effects, although the optimal therapeutic protocol, such as the timing and dose of cells, is not known. This therapy, intravenous infusion of autologous UCB cells (UCBCs), is considered to have the lowest risk in clinical translation for infants with brain injury [20].

1.2.2 Clinical Use of Cell Therapy with Umbilical Cord Blood

Blood transfusion is the oldest cell therapy for mankind. Hematopoietic stem cell (HSC) transplantation, i.e., BM transplantation, is the first cell therapy to use the regenerative property of stem cells and a well-established standard therapy for patients with leukemia and other malignant diseases. BM transplantation exerts benefits for mitigating neurodegenerative progress in some inborn errors of metabolism, such as Hurler's disease and adrenoleukodystrophy [21–23]. UCB contains a high concentration of HSCs; hence UCB transplantation is an excellent alternative for BM transplantation. UCB transplantation favorably alters the disease progression of some inborn errors of metabolism as well [24, 25]. The beneficial effect of HSC transplantation is primarily through enzyme replacement by the donor cells. Healthy donor cells engraft in the recipient and continue to excrete the enzyme that is defective in the recipient. Although HSC transplantation involves the intravenous administration of HSCs, transfused cells enter the donor brain and survive for months [26]. In addition to enzyme replacement, HSC transplantation is considered to exert a benefit through its effect on the immune system, such as the effect of donor-derived microglia in the brain [27]. One case study suggests that donor gene material reaches neurons and that these neurons contain some proteins of the donor gene product [28]. Taking these findings together, intravenous administration of HSCs has effects on the brain through a couple of mechanisms other than the hematopoietic potency. In addition, there is no risk of tumorigenicity in either UCB or BM transplantation.

1.3 Current Status of Cell Therapies for Brain Injury

Among the variety of cell types to be used for cell therapies, autologous UCBCs are the most feasible; the collection of the cells is totally noninvasive, and no ethical issues are involved as UCBs are usually discarded directly after birth. The safety and feasibility of intravenous infusion of cryopreserved autologous UCB have been reported in a study in children with neurological disorders, most of whom had CP [29]. Among 184 study participants, three patients experienced infusion reaction, which resolved after discontinuation of the infusion and medical therapy. No other adverse events were reported during the 12-month follow-up. Supported with positive results of systemic administration of hUCBCs in preclinical studies on neonatal encephalopathy, several institutions in several countries have started applying UCB transfusion for children with brain injury of non-metabolic origin.

1.3.1 Systemic Administration of UCBCs for Chronic Brain Injury

The chronic phase of brain injury is an easier target to treat with cell therapy compared with the acute phase of brain injury especially when the injury is sudden onset as in neonatal encephalopathy. Hence, CP has been the main target of UCBC therapy thus far. CP is a group of permanent disorders affecting motor development and posture resulting from various ischemic brain injuries that occur during the prenatal or neonatal period, of which neonatal HIE is the most conspicuous cause. Nearly 20 clinical trials are listed on the website of the US National Institute of Health (ClinicalTrials.gov) as a cell therapy for CP and related diseases (Table 1.1). Approximately half of the trials use UCB and the other half use cells derived from BM.

Of the 20 trials, 11 trials from six research groups use UCBCs. Only one of those trials has published the results thus far (NCT01193660) [30]. NCT01193660 is a randomized trial with 96 participants conducted at CHA University in South Korea. HLA-matched allogeneic UCB containing $>3 \times 10^7$/kg total nucleated cells (TNCs) was intravenously administered to children with CP along with erythropoietin and immunosuppressive treatment. Compared with the control group and the group treated with erythropoietin only, the UCB-treated group had significantly higher scores on the Gross Motor Performance Measure and Bayley II Mental and Motor Scales at 6 months. The incidence of serious adverse events did not differ between groups. The same group compared allogeneic (three patients) and autologous (four

Table 1.1 Review of clinical trials of chronic phase treatment in children with cerebral palsy and the related diseases

		ClinicalTrials.gov			Participants					Cell				
		Identifier	Phase	Status	Diagnosis	Number	Age	Arms	Randomization	Source	Type	Dose	Route	Location
1	A	NCT01019733	NA	Completed, published	CP with perinatal HI	18	2–5 year	1	–	Auto	BM-TNC	5-50 × 10^8	i.t. and i.v.	Mexico
2	A	NCT02231242	II	Recruiting	Quadriplegic CP	60	7–9 year	2	+	Auto	BM-TNC	NA	i.t.	Mexico
3		NCT01072370	I, II	Recruiting	CP	40	1–12 year	2	+	Auto	UCB-MNC	>1 × 10^7/kg	i.v.	USA[b]
4	B	NCT01147653	II	Recruiting	Spastic CP	120	1–6 year	2	+	Auto	UCB	>1 × 10^7/kg	i.v.	USA[c]
5	B	NCT02599207	I	Recruiting	CP	15	12 month–6 year	2	–	allo	UCB[a]	>2.5 × 10^7/kg	i.v.	USA[c]
6	C	NCT01193660	NA	Completed, published	CP	96	10 month–10 year	3	+	allo	UCB	>3 × 10^7/kg	i.v.	Korea
7	C	NCT01528436	II	Completed	CP	37	6 month–20 year	2	+	allo	UCB	NA	i.v. or i.a.	Korea
8	C	NCT01639404	NA	Completed	CP	17	6 month–20 year	1	–	allo	UCB	NA	i.v. or i.a.	Korea
9	C	NCT01991145	NA	Recruiting	CP	120	10 month–6 year	4	+	allo	UCB	NA	i.v.	Korea
10	C	NCT02025972	NA	Recruiting	CP	18	<15 year	1	–	allo	UCB-TNC	>3 × 10^/kg	NA	Korea
11	D	NCT01404663	I	Completed	Spastic quadriplegic CP	12	4–12 year	1	–	Auto	BM CD133+	NA	i.t.	Iran
12	D	NCT01763255	I, II	Completed	Spastic quadriplegic CP	8	4–12 year	2	+	NA	BM CD133+	NA	i.t.	Iran
13	E	NCT01832454	II, III	Recruiting	CP	100	3–5 year	1	–	Auto	BM-MNC	1 × 10^8	i.t.	India

		ClinicalTrials.gov			Participants					Cell				
		Identifier	Phase	Status	Diagnosis	Number	Age	Arms	Randomization	Source	Type	Dose	Route	Location
14	E	NCT01834664	I/II	Recruiting	Ataxic CP	100	15–70 year	1	–	Auto	BM-MNC	1×10^6	i.t.	India
15		NCT01929434	III	Before recruiting	CP	300	1–14 year	3	+	NA	UCB-MSC	NA	i.t.	China
16	F	NCT01978821	I	Completed	CP	40	17 month–22 year	1	–	Auto	BM-MNC	NA	NA	India
17	F	NCT02241395	I	Recruiting	CP	500	6 month–35 year	1	–	Auto	BM-MNC	NA	NA	India
18		NCT01988584	II	Recruiting	CP	30	2–10 year	3	+	Auto	UCB or BM-MNC	NA	i.v.	USA[d]
19		NCT02460484	I/II	Recruiting	Perinatal arterial stroke	10	6 week–6 year	1	–	Auto	UCB	NA	Infusion	USA[e]
20		NCT02574923	II	Recruiting	CP caused by O_2 deprivation	30	2–15 year	1	–	Auto	BM-MNC	NA	i.t.	Vietnam
		(NCT02569775)	Almost identical with NCT02574923											

A, B, C, the same letter of the alphabet indicates the same institute, *NA* information not available, *CP* cerebral palsy, *HI* hypoxia-ischemia, *Auto* autologous, *allo* allogeneic, *BM* bone marrow, *TNC* total nucleated cell *UCB* umbilical cord blood, *MNC* mononuclear cell, *MSC* mesenchymal stem cell, *i.v.* intravenous, *i.t.* intrathecal *i.a.* intra-arterial

[a]HLA-matched vs mismatched

[b]Georgia Regents University

[c]Duke University

[d]University of Texas Health Science Center, Houston

[e]Florida Hospital

patients) UCB transplantation in children with CP [31]. The allogeneic transplantation showed a better outcome than autologous transplantation.

Among the remaining ten trials, one trial (NCT01988584) uses either autologous UCB or BM-MNCs, three other trials (NCT01072370, NCT01147653, NCT02460484) use autologous UCB, five trials (NCT01528436, NCT01639404, NCT01991145, NCT02025972, NCT02599207) use allogeneic UCB, and one trial (NCT01929434) does not specify the source of UCB. Cells are administered intravenously in many of the trials but intra-arterially or intrathecally in some trials. NCT01929434 is the only phase III trial among them; the rest of them are either phase I or II trials. Regarding the cell types used, MSCs are used in a single trial (NCT01929434), MNCs are used in some trials (NCT01988584, NCT01072370), and the cell type used is not described in other trials.

Apart from the clinical studies listed on ClinicalTrials.gov, there are a few case reports of cell therapies in infants with brain injury. Jensen and Hamelmann reported the case of a boy with HI brain injury due to cardiac arrest at 2 years of age [32]. The boy received autologous intravenous UCB transfusion 9 weeks after the cardiac arrest. He demonstrated remarkable neurofunctional recovery from a vegetative state during the 2 months after the cell therapy. Jansen and Hamelmann attribute the recovery to the cell therapy. A pilot study of the intravenous infusion of autologous UCB was conducted in 20 children with CP with no control group [33]. Five children showed more improvements in neurodevelopmental evaluations than would normally be expected during the 6-month period after the infusion. Clinical studies using cells derived other than from either UCB or BM are limited. A randomized control trial of allogeneic transplantations of olfactory ensheathing cells (OECs) in 33 children with CP has been reported [34]. OECs were isolated from an aborted human fetal olfactory bulb, and the cells were injected into the frontal lobe of the patients. The OEC-treated children showed better Gross Motor Function Measure score than the controls. Although these results seem promising, it is difficult to interpret the efficacy as they are a case report and a clinical trial with no control group or with a small sample size.

1.3.2 Systemic Administration of UCBCs for Acute Brain Injury

Treating sudden onset diseases during their acute phase is difficult. Cells that require a preparation process with cell culture cannot be used during the acute phase, as cell culture takes from days to weeks. Hence, when culture work is required to prepare them, cells should be allogeneically prepared in advance (off-the-shelf). Autologous cells are advantageous over allogeneic cells in many respects; autologous cells have no or minimal risks on immune reactions and virus infections, no ethical issues related to the donors, and no shortage of donors. BM cells are a feasible autologous cell source for acute treatment in children and adults. However, collecting BM cells from a sick newborn is relatively invasive. In contrast, the collection of UCB is totally noninvasive for a newborn and his or her mother. For these reasons, autologous UCB is the most feasible cell source of autologous cells for treating acute onset diseases during the acute phase.

1.3.2.1 Clinical Trials of Systemic Administration of UCBCs for Acute Brain Injury

Seven clinical trials are listed on ClinicalTrials.gov as trials for newborns with neonatal encephalopathy to the best of our knowledge: NCT00593242, NCT02612155NCT01506258, NCT01649648, NCT02256618, NCT02434965, NCT02605018 (NCT02551003 seems identical to NCT02605018), and NCT02612155 (Table 1.2). All of them use autologous UCB. The registration websites of five of the trials do not specify the cell type used, most of which are assumed to be volume-reduced whole nucleated cells. The remaining two trials use either UCB $CD34^{+}$ cells or UCB along with placenta-derived stem cells. Almost all of them are administered intravenously; two trials do not specify the administration route. Apart from one trial, in which cells are infused up to 7 days after birth, cells are administered within a few days after birth.

Only NCT00593242 (principal investigator, Dr. Cotten at Duke University, USA) has been completed, and the results have been published [35]. Cotten and colleagues enrolled 23 infants treated with hypothermia for HIE and intravenously infused non-cryopreserved volume- and red blood cell-reduced UCBCs: up to four doses (up to two doses in the current protocol), ~72 postnatal hours (~48 postnatal hours in the current protocol), and the mean number of cells after processing 4.1×10^{8} cells/patient. No significant infusion reactions were noted. One-year neurodevelopmental outcomes were assessed with Bayley III, and 72% of UCBC treated infants had Bayley scores ≥85. Of infants who did not have available UCB and received standard treatments including hypothermia during the study period, 41% had Bayley scores ≥85. Of note, 26% of UCBC-treated infants were outborn (transported from an outside hospital after delivery), while 88% of infants with standard treatment were outborn. As outborn infants generally tend to have poorer outcome than inborn infants, caution should be exercised in interpreting the benefit of UCBCs. Nevertheless, the trial suggests that autologous UCBC infusion therapy for neonatal HIE is safe and feasible and may improve the outcome.

One of the seven trials is being conducted by us in Japan (NCT02256618, principal investigator, Dr. Shintaku at Osaka City University); our protocol is similar to the one at Duke University.

1.3.2.2 Our Clinical Trial of Systemic Administration of UCBCs for Acute Brain Injury

We, Neonatal Encephalopathy Consortium Japan, are currently conducting a phase I trial named "Autologous cord blood cell therapy for neonatal encephalopathy" (NCT02256618). This is a pilot study for testing the feasibility and safety of UCBC

Table 1.2 Review of clinical trials of acute phase treatment in newborns with neonatal encephalopathy

		ClinicalTrials.gov			Participants				Cell					
		Identifier	Phase	Status	Diagnosis	Number	Arms	Randomization	Source	Type	Dose	Timing	Route	Location
1	A	NCT00593242	I	Completed, published	HIE (a)	23	1	–	Auto	UCB[b]	1–5 × 10^7 × 4	~72 h	i.v.	USA[c]
2	A	NCT02612155	II	Not yet recruiting	HIE	160	2	+	Auto	UCB[b]	NA	~48 h?	i.v.	USA[c]
3		NCT01506258	NA	NA	Asphyxia[a]	20	2	–	Auto	UCB CD34+	NA	~48 h	i.v.	Mexico
4		NCT01649648	I	Recruiting	HIE (c)	10	1	–	Auto	UCB	NA	~3 day	NA	Singapore
5		NCT02256618	I	Recruiting	HIE	6	1	–	Auto	UCB[b]	NA	~72 h	i.v.	Japan
6		NCT02434965	II	Not yet recruiting	HIE	20	1	–	Auto	HPDSC + UCB	NA	~7 day	Infusion	USA[d]
7		NCT02605018	I/II	Not yet recruiting	NE	60	2	+	Auto	UCB	NA	~72 h	i.v.	China
		(NCT 02551003)	Almost identical with NCT02605018											

A The same letter of the alphabet indicates the same institute, *NA* information not available, *HIE* hypoxic-ischemic encephalopathy, *auto* autologous, *UCB* umbilical cord blood, *HPDSC* human placenta-derived stem cells, *MNC* mononuclear cell, *i.v.* intravenous

[a]37–42 week, Apger <5 at 5 min, UCB pH <7.0, signs of HIE

[b]Volume reduced

[c]Duke Univ.

[d]New York Medical College

therapy in infants with neonatal HIE; the study is an open-label single group assignment. If a neonate is born with signs and symptoms of moderate to severe encephalopathy and meets the criteria for therapeutic hypothermia, the neonate is considered for entry of this clinical study; inclusion and exclusion criteria for the study are set in line with those of therapeutic hypothermia for term newborns with HIE (Table 1.3). Estimated enrollment is six cases. To make sure that UCB is properly collected without contamination, we exclude outborn infants from the trial. If an infant is born with severe asphyxia, the UCB is collected directly after the birth from an umbilical cord vein with special care to avoid contamination. We obtain parental consent before collecting UCB. UCB is volume- and red blood cell-reduced by centrifugation in a closed system using an automated machine named Sepax (Biosafe Inc. Switzerland). The volume- and red blood cell-reduced UCB contains all sorts of nucleated cells, including a variety of stem cells such as $CD34^+$ hematopoietic stem/endothelial progenitor cells. The processed UCB is divided into three doses and stored at 4 °C until use. The cell dose is not adjusted. The total amount of UCB collected is used after the abovementioned simple centrifugation. Estimated cell doses administered would be approximately 6×10^8 cells/newborn. If the total amount of UCB is less than 40 mL, the newborn shall not be enrolled in the trial

Table 1.3 Entry criteria for our clinical trial; autologous cord blood cell therapy for neonatal encephalopathy

Inclusion criteria
Infants are eligible if they meet all the following inclusion criteria except ④
1. ≥36 weeks gestation
2. Either a 10-min Apgar score ≤ 5, continued need for resuscitation for at least 10 min, or severe acidosis, defined as pH <7.0
Or base deficit ≥ 16 mmol/L in a sample of umbilical cord blood or any blood during the first hour after birth
3. Moderate to severe encephalopathy (Sarnat II to III)
4. A moderately or severely abnormal background amplitude-integrated EEG (aEEG) voltage or seizures identified by aEEG, if monitored
5. Up to 24 h of age
6. Autologous umbilical cord blood available to infuse within 3 days after birth
7. A person with parental authority must have given consent for the study
Exclusion criteria
1. Known major congenital anomalies, such as chromosomal anomalies, heart diseases
2. Major intracranial hemorrhage identified by brain ultrasonography or computed tomography
3. Severe growth restriction, with birth weight less than 1800 g
4. Severe infectious disease, such as sepsis
5. Hyperkalemia
6. Outborn infants (infants born at hospitals other than the study sites)
7. Volume of collected cord blood <40 mL
8. Infants judged critically ill and unlikely to benefit from neonatal intensive care by the attending neonatologist

aEEG amplitude-integrated EEG

because the automated UCB process may not be reliable if the volume to be processed were less than 40 mL. We examined the quality of the processed and noncryopreserved UCB using UCB collected from volunteers before commencement of this trial. At 72 h after the processing, there was no growth of bacteria or increase in potassium, and cell viability was well maintained. We obtain written informed consent from the parent(s) twice; first, when we consider the newborn with HIE meets the entry criteria after the initial assessment, which is normally a few hours after the birth, and, second, before the first administration of UCBC treatment for the newborn.

Autologous volume-reduced cord blood cells are administered intravenously at 12–24, 36–48, and 60–72 h after birth. Circulatory and respiratory status is closely monitored during and after the cell treatment. The primary outcome measure is the rate of adverse events. The combined rate of three adverse events at 30 days of age, death, continuous respiratory support, and continuous use of vasopressor, will be compared between the neonates with cell therapy and those with conventional therapy including hypothermia. The secondary outcome measure is efficacy. Neuroimaging at 12 months of age and neurodevelopmental function measured with Bayley III at 18 months of age will be compared between the cell recipients and neonates with conventional therapy. The infants will be followed for safety and neurodevelopmental outcome up to 10 years of age.

1.3.3 Systemic Administration of UCBCs for Brain Injury Associated with Preterm Birth

To the best of our knowledge, as few as one clinical trial (NCT01121328) is listed on ClinicalTrials.gov with respect to cell treatment for brain injury associated with preterm birth. The clinical trial focuses on premature infants born less than 34 weeks of gestation. Autologous UCB-MNCs are infused in the first 14 days after birth.

1.3.4 Issues to be Considered for UCBC Therapies

All those trials but one are small nonrandomized ones; therefore the efficacy of the cell therapies would not be known. The group led by Cotten is preparing a phase II clinical trial (NCT02612155) with an estimated enrollment of 160 cases.

The properties of hUCBCs may be altered by several factors, such as the gestational age and perinatal asphyxia [36, 37]. For example, Aly et al. reported that although the UCB-MNC count does not differ between healthy term newborns and term newborns with perinatal asphyxia, neuronal differentiation of hUCB-MSCs is more pronounced in the cells derived from newborns with asphyxia [38]. Lymphocyte counts are elevated in term infants with HIE, although the counts rapidly normalized [39]. The apoptosis of neutrophils is impaired in cord blood compared with adult peripheral blood, and the apoptosis is reduced by hypoxia [40]. Those alterations may become beneficial or detrimental to infants receiving UCB therapy.

Autologous UCBC treatment is the most feasible cell therapy for neonates with encephalopathy during the acute phase. Although the therapy has the lowest risk for clinical use, there are some drawbacks. The following two issues are critical. Firstly, autologous UCB may be difficult to collect in an urgent situation. Secondly, the risk of bacterial contamination is not negligible as the UCB is not cryopreserved for days, especially when a neonate is born via vaginal delivery at a small hospital with limited medical staff.

1.4 Conclusion

A growing number of preclinical studies suggest that systemic administration of UCBCs has the potential for ameliorating infant brain injury even when the treatment is started days after the insult. As having the lowest risk in clinical use for sick newborns, intravenous administration of autologous UCBCs without cell sorting and cell culturing has been tried in many institutions in several countries. There is, however, a paucity of preclinical data on the optimal treatment protocol for neonatal encephalopathy. Rigorous preclinical studies are needed to optimize the protocol as well as to clarify the mechanisms of action. At the same time, many patients and their parents are desperately seeking opportunities to receive cell therapies, as the current therapies for neonatal encephalopathy and its neurological sequelae offer limited hope. We believe it is important to proceed with clinical trials promptly under monitoring by the regulatory authorities.

References

1. Dammann O, Ferriero D, Gressens P. Neonatal encephalopathy or hypoxic-ischemic encephalopathy? Appropriate terminology matters. Pediatr Res. 2011;70:1–2.
2. Volpe JJ. Neonatal encephalopathy: an inadequate term for hypoxic-ischemic encephalopathy. Ann Neurol. 2012;72:156–66.
3. van Handel M, Swaab H, de Vries LS, Jongmans MJ. Long-term cognitive and behavioral consequences of neonatal encephalopathy following perinatal asphyxia: a review. Eur J Pediatr. 2007;166:645–54.
4. Lindstrom K, Lagerroos P, Gillberg C, Fernell E. Teenage outcome after being born at term with moderate neonatal encephalopathy. Pediatr Neurol. 2006;35:268–74.
5. Gluckman PD, Wyatt JS, Azzopardi D, Ballard R, Edwards AD, Ferriero DM, et al. Selective head cooling with mild systemic hypothermia after neonatal encephalopathy: multicentre randomised trial. Lancet. 2005;365:663–70.
6. Shankaran S, Laptook AR, Ehrenkranz RA, Tyson JE, McDonald SA, Donovan EF, et al. National Institute of Child H, Human Development Neonatal Research Network. Whole-body hypothermia for neonates with hypoxic-ischemic encephalopathy. N Engl J Med. 2005;353:1574–84.

7. O'Collins VE, Macleod MR, Donnan GA, Horky LL, van der Worp BH, Howells DW. 1,026 experimental treatments in acute stroke. Ann Neurol. 2006;59:467–77.
8. Castillo-Melendez M, Yawno T, Jenkin G, Miller SL. Stem cell therapy to protect and repair the developing brain: a review of mechanisms of action of cord blood and amnion epithelial derived cells. Front Neurosci. 2013;7:194.
9. Liao Y, Cotten M, Tan S, Kurtzberg J, Cairo MS. Rescuing the neonatal brain from hypoxic injury with autologous cord blood. Bone Marrow Transplant. 2013;48:890–900.
10. Bliss T, Guzman R, Daadi M, Steinberg GK. Cell transplantation therapy for stroke. Stroke. 2007;38:817–26.
11. Hess DC, Borlongan CV. Cell-based therapy in ischemic stroke. Expert Rev Neurother. 2008;8:1193–201.
12. Mendez-Otero R, de Freitas GR, Andre C, de Mendonca ML, Friedrich M, Oliveira-Filho J. Potential roles of bone marrow stem cells in stroke therapy. Regen Med. 2007;2:417–23.
13. Borlongan CV, Hadman M, Sanberg CD, Sanberg PR. Central nervous system entry of peripherally injected umbilical cord blood cells is not required for neuroprotection in stroke. Stroke. 2004;35:2385–9.
14. Sarnowska A, Braun H, Sauerzweig S, Reymann KG. The neuroprotective effect of bone marrow stem cells is not dependent on direct cell contact with hypoxic injured tissue. Exp Neurol. 2009;215:317–27.
15. Tsuji M, Johnston MV. Cell-based therapies in neonatal stroke. In: Hess DC, editor. Cell therapy for brain injury. Switzerland: Springer International; 2015. p. 321–49.
16. Elsayed MH, Hogan TP, Shaw PL, Castro AJ. Use of fetal cortical grafts in hypoxic-ischemic brain injury in neonatal rats. Exp Neurol. 1996;137:127–41.
17. Meier C, Middelanis J, Wasielewski B, Neuhoff S, Roth-Haerer A, Gantert M, et al. Spastic paresis after perinatal brain damage in rats is reduced by human cord blood mononuclear cells. Pediatr Res. 2006;59:244–9.
18. Yasuhara T, Hara K, Maki M, Mays RW, Deans RJ, Hess DC, et al. Intravenous grafts recapitulate the neurorestoration afforded by intracerebrally delivered multipotent adult progenitor cells in neonatal hypoxic-ischemic rats. J Cereb Blood Flow Metab. 2008;28:1804–10.
19. Tsuji M, Taguchi A, Ohshima M, Kasahara Y, Sato Y, Tsuda H, et al. Effects of intravenous administration of umbilical cord blood $CD34^+$ cells in a mouse model of neonatal stroke. Neuroscience. 2014;263:148–58.
20. Bennet L, Tan S, Van den Heuij L, Derrick M, Groenendaal F, van Bel F, et al. Cell therapy for neonatal hypoxia-ischemia and cerebral palsy. Ann Neurol. 2012;71:589–600.
21. Beam D, Poe MD, Provenzale JM, Szabolcs P, Martin PL, Prasad V, et al. Outcomes of unrelated umbilical cord blood transplantation for x-linked adrenoleukodystrophy. Biol Blood Marrow Transplant. 2007;13:665–74.
22. Peters C, Shapiro EG, Anderson J, Henslee-Downey PJ, Klemperer MR, Cowan MJ, et al. Hurler syndrome: II. Outcome of HLA-genotypically identical sibling and hla-haploidentical related donor bone marrow transplantation in fifty-four children. The storage disease collaborative study group. Blood. 1998;91:2601–8.
23. Peters C, Charnas LR, Tan Y, Ziegler RS, Shapiro EG, DeFor T, et al. Cerebral x-linked adrenoleukodystrophy: tThe international hematopoietic cell transplantation experience from 1982 to 1999. Blood. 2004;104:881–8.
24. Aldenhoven H, Kurtzberg J. Cord blood is the optimal graft source for the treatment of pediatric patients with lysosomal storage diseases: clinical outcomes and future directions. Cytotherapy. 2015;17:765–74.
25. Staba SL, Escolar ML, Poe M, Kim Y, Martin PL, Szabolcs P, et al. Cord-blood transplants from unrelated donors in patients with Hurler's syndrome. N Engl J Med. 2004;350:1960–9.
26. Mezey E, Key S, Vogelsang G, Szalayova I, Lange GD, Crain B. Transplanted bone marrow generates new neurons in human brains. Proc Natl Acad Sci U S A. 2003;100:1364–9.
27. Moser HW, Mahmood A. New insights about hematopoietic stem cell transplantation in adrenoleukodystrophy. Arch Neurol. 2007;64:631–2.

28. Schönberger S, Roerig P, Schneider DT, Reifenberger G, Gobel U, Gartner J. Genotype and protein expression after bone marrow transplantation for adrenoleukodystrophy. Arch Neurol. 2007;64:651–7.
29. Sun J, Allison J, McLaughlin C, Sledge L, Waters-Pick B, Wease S, et al. Differences in quality between privately and publicly banked umbilical cord blood units: a pilot study of autologous cord blood infusion in children with acquired neurologic disorders. Transfusion. 2010;50:1980–7.
30. Min K, Song J, Kang JY, Ko J, Ryu JS, Kang MS, et al. Umbilical cord blood therapy potentiated with erythropoietin for children with cerebral palsy: a double-blind, randomized, placebo-controlled trial. Stem Cells. 2013;31:581–91.
31. Bae SH, Lee HS, Kang MS, Strupp BJ, Chopp M, Moon J. The levels of pro-inflammatory factors are significantly decreased in cerebral palsy patients following an allogeneic umbilical cord blood cell transplant. Int J Stem Cells. 2012;5:31–8.
32. Jensen A, Hamelmann E. First autologous cell therapy of cerebral palsy caused by hypoxic-ischemic brain damage in a child after cardiac arrest-individual treatment with cord blood. Case Rep Transplant. 2013:951827.
33. Lee YH, Choi KV, Moon JH, Jun HJ, Kang HR, Oh SI, et al. Safety and feasibility of countering neurological impairment by intravenous administration of autologous cord blood in cerebral palsy. J Transl Med. 2012;10:58.
34. Chen L, Huang H, Xi H, Xie Z, Liu R, Jiang Z, et al. Intracranial transplant of olfactory ensheathing cells in children and adolescents with cerebral palsy: a randomized controlled clinical trial. Cell Transplant. 2010;19:185–91.
35. Cotten CM, Murtha AP, Goldberg RN, Grotegut CA, Smith PB, Goldstein RF, et al. Feasibility of autologous cord blood cells for infants with hypoxic-ischemic encephalopathy. J Pediatr. 2014;164:973–9. e971
36. Javed MJ, Mead LE, Prater D, Bessler WK, Foster D, Case J, et al. Endothelial colony forming cells and mesenchymal stem cells are enriched at different gestational ages in human umbilical cord blood. Pediatr Res. 2008;64:68–73.
37. Ligi I, Simoncini S, Tellier E, Vassallo PF, Sabatier F, Guillet B, et al. Sswitch toward angiostatic gene expression impairs the angiogenic properties of endothelial progenitor cells in low birth weight preterm infants. Blood. 2011;118:1699–709.
38. Aly H, Mohsen L, Badrawi N, Gabr H, Ali Z, Akmal D. Viability and neural differentiation of mesenchymal stem cells derived from the umbilical cord following perinatal asphyxia. J Perinatol. 2012;32:671–6.
39. Phelan JP, Korst LM, Ahn MO, Martin GI. Neonatal nucleated red blood cell and lymphocyte counts in fetal brain injury. Obstet Gynecol. 1998;91:485–9.
40. Hanna N, Graboski S, Laskin DL, Weinberger B. Effects of ibuprofen and hypoxia on neutrophil apoptosis in neonates. Biol Neonate. 2004;86:235–9.

Chapter 2
New Strategy of Clinical Studies for Premature Babies with Ischemic Brain Damage

Makoto Nabetani and Haruo Shintaku

Abstract In Japan, we started autologous cord blood therapy for newborns with HIE in 2014 (described in Chap. 1). Another research group started autologous cord blood therapy for patients with cerebral palsy in 2017. However, cerebral palsy is induced in nearly twice as many premature babies with IVH and PVL as that by term newborns with HIE (Touyama et al. Brain Dev 38:792–799, 2016; Koterazawa et al. No to Hattatsu 48:14–19, 2016; Glinianaia et al. Dev Med Child Neurol 59:864–870, 2017). Therefore, we are now promoting a new clinical study protocol of cell therapy for premature newborns with PVL or IVH.

Keywords Cell therapy · Periventricular leukomalacia · PVL · Intraventricular hemorrhage · IVH

2.1 Introduction

Clinical studies of regenerative medicine such as various types of stem cells, embryonic stem (ES) cells, and/or iPS cells have increased rapidly, and the number of clinical studies had exceeded 500 worldwide in 2016 [1]. However, hyperbole, distortion, and overselling of these regenerative medicines have also been reported in some journals [2]. Among these different strategies of cell therapies, the intravenous administration of UCB stem cell therapy could be the safest and most feasible because UCB has been used for hematopoietic stem cell transplantation in patients

M. Nabetani, M.D., Ph.D. (✉)
Department of Pediatrics, Yodogawa Christian Hospital, Higashiyodogawa-ku, 1-7-50, Osaka City, Japan
e-mail: a103111@ych.or.jp

H. Shintaku, M.D., Ph.D.
Department of Pediatrics, Osaka City University Graduate School of Medicine, Osaka-shi, Japan

© Springer Nature Singapore Pte Ltd. 2018

H. Shintaku et al. (eds.), *Cell Therapy for Perinatal Brain Injury*,
https://doi.org/10.1007/978-981-10-1412-3_2

with hematological diseases over several decades. Stem cells, obtained from umbilical cord blood, normally discarded after birth, are emerging as a safe and potentially effective therapy. Therefore, cell therapy using UCB has been expanded for novel applications. Recent reports have stated that the most common indication for UCB therapy is neurological diseases, including studies of cerebral palsy [3]. Other indications included diabetes mellitus, cardiac and vascular diseases, and hepatic diseases. Thirty-one studies administered total nucleated cells, mononuclear cells, or CD34+ cells, while 20 studies used cord blood-derived mesenchymal stromal cells. Eleven out of 46 studies described that cellular products used autologous products. They reported that 4/4 showed clinical benefit in cerebral palsy [4]. Furthermore, autologous UCB therapy has fewer ethical issues than allogenic UCB because autologous UCB has no possibility of rejection and no necessity of immune suppressive therapy to prevent rejection or GVHD. Therefore, autologous umbilical cord blood stem cell therapy could be the most feasible therapy for premature newborns with IVH or PVL. We are now challenging new project to investigate the feasibility and safety of autologous cord blood cell therapy for premature babies with IVH or PVL.

2.2 New Idea of Clinical Study Protocol

Major inclusion criteria included premature newborns who were born at 24–33 weeks old. The collection of baby cord blood cells is performed immediately after birth. The required volume of collected cord blood is over 15 mL. Separation is performed in cell processing center within 36 h of birth and returned to the hospital. The separated cord blood cells are administered intravenously within 36–72 h after birth (Fig. 2.1).

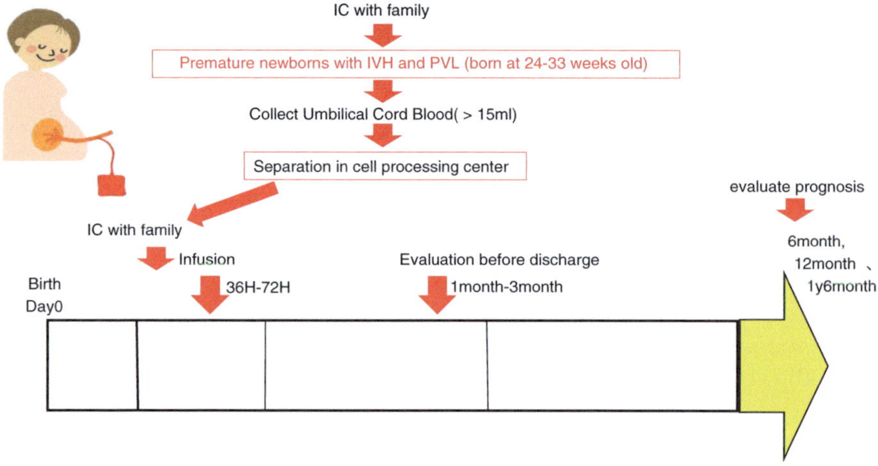

Fig. 2.1 New idea of cell therapy for premature newborns with IVH and PVL

2.3 Discussion

2.3.1 *Therapeutic Effect of UCB in a Hematopoietic Disease*

In 1982, Nakahata and Ogawa reported that umbilical cord blood contains hemopoietic colony-forming cells with extensive capability to generate mono- and multipotential hemopoietic progenitors [5]. Since then it has been confirmed that UBC also contains various rich stem cells such as hematopoietic stem cells, endothelial progenitor cells, and mesenchymal stromal cells.

CD34 surface antigen has been widely used as a marker of hematopoietic stem cells and endothelial progenitor cells. UCB contains about 0.3–2% CD34+ cells, while peripheral blood of an adult contains < 0.01% CD34+ cells [6–8].

Firstly, the therapeutic effects of UCB have been shown in hematological diseases, such as leukemia, Fanconi's anemia, and aplastic anemia, replacing the hematopoietic stem cells over the past few decades [9–14].

2.3.2 *Therapeutic Effect of UCB in Various Intractable Diseases*

In recent years, UCB has been identified as a source of endothelial stem/progenitor cells and has an effect on various intractable diseases including cerebral palsy, diabetes mellitus, cardiac and vascular diseases, and hepatic diseases. Various types of stem cells are possible sources of cell therapy for clinical applications especially for neurological diseases [15–17].

In 2004, Kurtzberg reported that allogeneic UCB has been used for patients with inherited metabolic disorders and neurodegenerative diseases, i.e., Hurler's syndrome and Krabbe's disease, with the aim of delivering the deficient enzyme through the stem cells. Seventeen of the 20 children were alive at the median point of 905 days after transplantation (event-free survival rate, 85%). Transplantation improved neurocognitive performance and decreased the somatic features of Hurler's syndrome. Cord blood from unrelated donors appears to be an excellent source of stem cells for transplantation in patients with Hurler's syndrome. Eleven asymptomatic newborns (age range, 12–44 days) and 14 symptomatic infants (age range, 142–352 days) with infantile Krabbe's disease underwent transplantation of UCB from unrelated donors after myeloablative chemotherapy. Transplantation of UCB from unrelated donors in newborns with infantile Krabbe's disease favorably altered the natural history of the disease. However, transplantation in babies after symptoms had developed did not result in substantive neurologic improvement [18, 19].

Also in 2004, Taguchi reported that CD 34+ cells are effective for brain damage after stroke and started phase 1–1/2a clinical studies for patients with stroke for the first time. Phase 1/2a study of CD 34+ cells therapy for 12 patients with stroke showed favorable neurologic recovery and improvement in cerebral blood flow and metabolism with no serious adverse events. In comparison with historical controls, patients receiving cell therapy had significantly better neurologic outcomes. The results indicated that intravenous transplantation of autologous bone marrow mononuclear cells is safe and feasible. Positive results and trends favoring neurologic recovery and improvement in cerebral blood flow and metabolism by cell therapy underscore the relevance of larger-scale, randomized controlled trials using this approach [20, 21].

2.3.3 Therapeutic Effect of UCB in Cerebral Palsy

In this chapter, we focus on the potential therapeutic effects of cell therapies especially UCB therapy for newborns with ischemic disease which has progressed dramatically over the past few decades. In 2006 Meier et al. reported the effectiveness of intraperitoneal infusion of UCB cells in rats with neonatal hypoxia [22]. Kurtzberg is conducting a phase 2 study for cerebral palsy by using autologous cord blood cells at Duke University in the USA. On the other hand, Cox et al. reported a feasibility study showing that autologous bone marrow mononuclear cells were logistically feasible and safe to prescribe intravenously for children suffering from head trauma within 48 h of incident in 2011 [23]. Wang and Sharma also started a clinical study using autologous bone marrow mononuclear cells for cerebral palsy patients in 2013 and 2015 [24, 25].

It was also reported that concomitant administration of allogeneic UCB and recombinant human erythropoietin may boost the efficacy of UCB, as it has neurotrophic effects. Thus, allogeneic UCB treatment might ameliorate motor and cognitive dysfunction in children with CP undergoing active rehabilitation, accompanied by structural and metabolic changes in the brain [26]. Subarachnoid placement of stem cells was performed for 180 cases with diplegia and quadriplegia after trauma in India. This was effective in 32% of patients with no short- and long-term adverse effects. In the long-term follow-up, functional indices improved in 57 (31.67%) patients, including 54 patients with traumatic paraplegia/quadriplegia, 2 with cerebral palsy, and 1 with viral encephalitis [27]. Recently, Mancias-Guerra started an open-label phase 1 trial to investigate the safety and tolerability of intrathecal delivery of autologous bone marrow nucleated cells in children with cerebral palsy [28].

2.3.4 Possibility of Therapeutic Effect of UCB in Premature Newborns with PVL and IVH

Rizk reported that the most common indication for UCB therapy was neurological diseases (25 studies), including studies of cerebral palsy (12 studies). Other indications included diabetes mellitus (nine studies), cardiac and vascular diseases (seven studies), and hepatic diseases (four studies). Most studies administered total nucleated cells, mononuclear cells, or CD34+ cells (31 studies), while 20 studies used cord blood-derived mesenchymal stem cells. Forty-six studies described cellular products obtained from allogeneic sources, while 11 studies used autologous products. They identified three indications where multiple prospective controlled studies have been published (4/4 studies reported clinical benefit in cerebral palsy, 1/3 studies reported benefit for cirrhosis, and 1/3 studies reported biochemical response in type 1 diabetes) [4]. Autologous UCB therapy has fewer ethical issues than allogenic UCB because autologous UCB has no possibility of rejection and no necessity of immune suppressive therapy to prevent rejection or GVHD. Autologous UCB stem cell therapy could be the most feasible therapy for premature newborns. Recent experimental and clinical reports have indicated that cord blood stem cell therapy might provide protective effect on hypoxic-ischemic brain damage by the process shown below:

1. Immunomodulation/anti-inflammatory action [29–31]
2. Reduction of apoptosis and oxidative stress [32–34]
3. Enhancement of regenerative process by secretion of various cytokines [35–38]
4. Enhancement of regenerative process by angiogenesis to better circulation of the brain [39–46]
5. Enhancement of regenerative process by neurogenesis [47–54]
6. However, clinical studies of autologous UCB stem cell therapy for premature newborns with IVH or PVL have not been published. We need to challenge the new clinical study to investigate feasibility and safety of autolougous UCB cell therapy for premature babies with IVH or PVL.

2.4 Conclusion

Autologous UCB stem cell therapy might be the most feasible therapy for premature newborns who were born at 24–33 weeks old. Further clarification is required on the feasibility and efficacy of cell therapy for premature newborn babies with IVH or PVL.

References

1. Kimmelman J, Hyun I, Benvenisty N, Caulfield T, Heslop HE, Murry CE, et al. Policy: global standards for stem cell research. Nature. 2016;533:311–3.
2. Caulfield T, Sipp D, Murry CE, Daley GQ, Kimmelman J. Confronting stem cell hype. Science. 2016;352:776–7.
3. Bennet L, Tan S, Gunn AJ, Derrick M, Groenendaal F, van Bel F, et al. Cell therapy for neonatal hypoxia–ischemia and cerebral palsy. Ann Neurol. 2012;71:589–600.
4. Rizk M, Aziz J, Allan DS, Allan DS. Cell-based therapy using umbilical cord blood for novel indications in regenerative therapy and immune modulation: an updated systematic scoping review of the literature. Biol Blood Marrow Transplant. 2017;23:1607–13.

5. Nakahata T, Ogawa M. Hemopoietic colony-forming cells in umbilical cord blood with extensive capability to generate mono- and multipotential hemopoietic progenitors. J Clin Invest. 1982;70:1324–8.
6. Murohara T, Ikeda H, Duan J, Shintani S, Sasaki K, Eguchi H, et al. Transplanted cord blood-derived endothelial precursor cells augment postnatal neovascularization. J Clin Invest. 2000;105:1527–36.
7. Sun J, Allison J, McLaughlin C, Sledge L, Waters-Pick B, Wease S, et al. Differences in quality between privately and publicly banked umbilical cord blood units: a pilot study of autologous cord blood infusion in children with acquired neurologic disorders. Transfusion. 2010;50:1980–7.
8. Michejda M. Which stem cells should be used for transplantation? Fetal Diagn Ther. 2004;19:2–8.
9. Auerbach AD, Liu Q, Ghosh R, Pollack MS, Douglas GW, Broxmeyer HE. Prenatal identification of potential donors for umbilical cord blood transplantation for Fanconi anemia. Transfusion. 1990;30(8):682–7.
10. Gluckman E, Rocha V, Boyer-Chammard A, Locatelli F, Arcese W, Pasquini R, et al. Eurocord transplant group and the European blood and marrow transplantation group. Outcome of cord-blood transplantation from related and unrelated donors. N Engl J Med. 1997;337(6):373–81.
11. Kurtzberg J, Laughlin M, Graham ML, Smith C, Olson JF, Halperin EC, et al. Placental blood as a source of hematopoietic stem cells for transplantation into unrelated recipients. N Engl J Med. 1996;335(3):157–66.
12. Herr AL, Kabbara N, Bonfim CM, Teira P, Locatelli F, Tiedemann K, et al. Long-term follow-up and factors influencing outcomes after related HLA-identical cord blood transplantation for patients with malignancies: an analysis on behalf of Eurocord-EBMT. Blood. 2010;116(11):1849–56.
13. Hassall OW, Thitiri J, Fegan G, Hamid F, Mwarumba S, Denje D, et al. Safety and efficacy of allogeneic umbilical cord red blood cell transfusion for children with severe anaemia in a Kenyan hospital: an open-label single-arm trial. Lancet Haematol. 2015;2(3):e101–7.
14. Hassall O, Bedu-Addo G, Adarkwa M, Danso K, Bates I. Umbilical-cord blood for transfusion in children with severe anaemia in under-resourced countries. Lancet. 2003;361:678–9.
15. Lindvall O, Kokaia Z. Stem cells for the treatment of neurological disorders. Nature. 2006;441:1094–6.
16. Sato Y, Oohira A. Chondroitin sulfate, a major niche substance of neural stem cells, and cell transplantation therapy of neurodegeneration combined with niche modification. Curr Stem Cell Res Ther. 2009;4:200–9.
17. Li J, Yawno T, Sutherland A, Loose J, Nitsos I, Bischof R, et al. Preterm white matter brain injury is prevented by early administration of umbilical cord blood cells. Exp Neuro. 2016;283:179–87.
18. Staba SL, Escolar ML, Poe M, Kim Y, Kurtzberg J, Martin PL, et al. Cord-blood transplants from unrelated donors in patients with Hurler's syndrome. N Engl J Med. 2004;350(19):1960–9.
19. Escolar ML, Poe MD, Provenzale JM, Richards KC, Allison J, Wood S, et al. Transplantation of umbilical-cord blood in babies with infantile Krabbe's disease. N Engl J Med. 2005;352(20):2069–81.
20. Akihiko Soma T, Tanaka H, Kanda T, Nishimura H, Yoshikawa H, et al. Administration of CD34+ cells after stroke enhances neurogenesis via angiogenesis in a mouse model. J Clin Invest. 2004;414:330–8.
21. Taguchi A, Sakai C, Soma T, et al. Intravenous autologous bone marrow mononuclear cell transplantation for stroke: phase1/2A clinical trial in a homogeneous group of stroke patients. Stem Cells Dev. 2015;24(19):2207–18.
22. Meier C, Middelanis J, Neuhoff S, Roth-Haerer A, Gantert M. Spastic paresis after perinatal brain damage in rats is reduced by human cord blood mononuclear cells. Pediatr Res. 2006;59:244–9.
23. Cox CS Jr, Baumgartner JE, Gee A, Worth LL, Walker PA, Shah SK, et al. Autologous bone marrow mononuclear cell therapy for severe traumatic brain injury in children. Neurosurgery. 2011;68:588–600.

24. Wang X, Cheng H, Hua Y, Yang J, Dai G, Zhang Z, et al. Effects of bone marrow mesenchymal stromal cells on gross motor function measure scores of children with cerebral palsy: a preliminary clinical study. Cytotherapy. 2013;15:1549–62.
25. Sharma A, Sane H, Badhe P, Gokulchandran N, Kulkarni P, Gandhi S, et al. A clinical study of autologous bone marrow mononuclear cells for cerebral palsy patients: a new frontier. Stem Cells Int. 2015;2015:905874.
26. Min K, Song J, Kim M, Ko J, Ryu JS, Kang MS. Umbilical cord blood therapy potentiated with erythropoietin for children with cerebral palsy: a double-blind, randomized, placebo-controlled trial. Stem Cells. 2013;31:581–91.
27. Mehta T, Feroz A, Trivedi H, Vanikar A, Shah V, Trivedi H. Subarachnoid placement of stem cells in neurological disorders. Transplant Proc. 2008;40:1145–7.
28. Mancías-Guerra C, Marroquín-Escamilla AR, Gómez-Almaguer D, Villarreal-Martínez L, Jaime-Pérez JC, García-Rodríguez F. Safety and tolerability of intrathecal delivery of autologous bone marrow nucleated cells in children with cerebral palsy: an open-label phase I trial. Cytotherapy. 2014;16:810–20.
29. Rosenkranz K, Tenbusch M, May C, Marcus K, Meier C. Changes in Interleukin-1 alpha serum levels after transplantation of umbilical cord blood cells in a model of perinatal hypoxic– ischemic brain damage. Ann Anat. 2013;195:122–7.
30. Wasielewski B, Jensen A, Roth-Härer A, Dermietzel R, Meier C. Neuroglial activation and Cx43 expression are reduced upon transplantation of human umbilical cord blood cells after perinatal hypoxic–ischemic injury. Brain Res. 2012;1487:39–53.
31. Paton MCB, McDonald CA, Allison BJ, Fahey MC, Jenkin G, Miller SL, et al. Perinatal brain injury as a consequence of preterm birth and intrauterine inflammation: designing targeted stem cell therapies. Front Neurosci. 2017;11:200.
32. Rosenkranz K, Kumbruch S, Marcus K, Marschner K, Dermietzel R. Transplantation of human umbilical cord blood cells mediated beneficial effects on apoptosis, angiogenesis and neuronal survival after hypoxic–ischemic brain injury in rats. Cell Tissue Res. 2012;348:429–38.
33. Hattori T, Sato Y, Kondo T, Ichinohashi Y, Sugiyama Y, Yamamoto M, et al. Administration of umbilical cord blood cells transiently decreased hypoxic-ischemic brain injury in neonatal rats. Dev Neurosci. 2015;37:95–104.
34. Pimentel-Coelho PM, Magalhaes ES, Lopes LM, LC DA, Santiago MF, Mendez-Otero R. Human cord blood transplantation in a neonatal rat model of hypoxic–ischemic brain damage: functional outcome related to neuroprotection in the striatum. Stem Cells Dev. 2010;19:351–8.
35. Yoshihara T, Taguchi A, Matsuyama T, Shimizu Y, Kikuchi-Taura A, Soma T, Stern DM, et al. Increase in circulating CD34positive cells in patients with angiographic evidence of moyamoya-like vessels. J Cereb Blood Flow Metab. 2008;28:1086–9.
36. Rosenkranz K, Kumbruch S, Kumbruch S, Lebermann K, Marschner K, Jensen A, Dermietzel R, et al. The chemokine SDF-1/CXCL12 contributes to the ‘homing’ of umbilical cord blood cells to a hypoxic–ischemic lesion in the rat brain. J Neurosci Res. 2010;88:1223–33.
37. Yasuhara T, Hara K, Maki M, Xu L, Yu G, Ali MM, et al. Mannitol facilitates neurotrophic factor up-regulation and behavioural recovery in neonatal hypoxic-ischaemic rats with human umbilical cord blood grafts. J Cell Mol Med. 2010;14:914–21.
38. Majka M, Janowska-Wieczorek A, Ratajczak J, Ehrenman K, Pietrzkowski Z, Kowalska MA, et al. Numerous growth factors, cytokines, and chemokines are secreted by human CD34+cells, myeloblasts, erythroblasts, and megakaryoblasts and regulate normal hematopoiesis in an autocrine/paracrine manner. Blood. 2001;97:3705–085.
39. Taguchi A, Matsuyama T, Moriwaki H, Hayashi T, Hayashida K, Nagatsuka K, et al. Circulating CD34-positive cells provide an index of cerebrovascular function. Circulation. 2004;109:2972–5.
40. Taguchi A, Soma T, Tanaka H, Kanda T, Nishimura H, Yoshikawa H, et al. Administration of CD34+ cells after stroke enhances neurogenesis via angiogenesis in a mouse model. J Clin Invest. 2004;414:330–8.

41. Asahara T, Murohara T, Sullivan A, Silver M, van der Zee R, Li T, et al. Isolation of putative progenitor endothelial cells for angiogenesis. Science. 1997;275:964–7.
42. Asahara T, Masuda H, Takahashi T, Kalka C, Pastore C, Silver M, et al. Bone marrow origin of endothelial progenitor cells responsible for postnatal vasculogenesis in physiological and pathological neovascularization. Cir Res. 1999;85:221–8.
43. Jin K, Zhu Y, Sun Y, Mao XO, Xie L, Greenberg DA. Vascular endothelial growth factor (VEGF) stimulates neurogenesis in vitro and in vivo. Proc Natl Acad Sci USA. 2002;99:11946–50.
44. Kawamoto A, Gwon HC, Iwaguro H, Yamaguchi JI, Uchida S, Masuda H, et al. Therapeutic potential of ex vivo expanded endothelial progeny cells for myocardial ischemia. Circulation. 2001;103:634–7.
45. Nakatomi H, Kuriu T, Okabe S, Yamamoto S, Hatano O, Kawahara N, et al. Regeneration of hippocampal pyramidal neurons after ischemic brain injury by recruitment of endogenous neuronal progenitors. Cell. 2002;110:429–41.
46. Drago J, Murphy M, Carroll SM, Harvey RP, Bartlett PF. Fibroblasts growth factor mediated proliferations of central nervous system precursors depends on endogenous production of insulin-like growth factor 1. Proc Natl Acad Sci U S A. 1991;88:2199–203.
47. Kasahara Y, Yamahara K, Yamahara K, Soma T, Stern DM, Nakagomi T, Matsuyama T, et al. Transplantation of hematopoietic stem cells: intra-arterial versus intravenous administration impacts stroke outcomes in a murine model. Transl Res. 2016;176:69–80.
48. Felling RJ, Snyder MJ, Snyder MJ, Romanko MJ, Rothstein RP, Ziegler AN. Neural stem/progenitor cells participate in the regenerative response to perinatal hypoxia/ischemia. J Neurosci. 2006;26:4359–69.
49. Eglitis MA, Mezey E. Hematopoietic cells differentiate into both microglia and macroglia in the brains of adult mice. Proc Natl Acad Sci U S A. 1997;94:4080–5.
50. Mezey E, Key S, Vogelsang G, Lange GD, Crain B. Transplanted bone marrow generates new neurons in human brains. Proc Natl Acad Sci U S A. 2003;100:1364–9.
51. Li Y, Adomat H, Guns ET, Hojabrpour P, Duronio V, Curran TA, et al. Identification of a hematopoietic cell dedifferentiation-inducing factor. J Cell Physiol. 2016;231:1350–63.
52. Chen SH, Wang JJ, Chen CH, Chang HK, Lin MT, Chang FM, et al. Umbilical cord blood-derived $CD34^+$ cells improve outcomes of traumatic brain injury in rats by stimulating angiogenesis and neurogenesis. Cell Transplant. 2014;23:959–79.
53. Davoust N, Vuaillat C, Cavillon G, Domenget C, Hatterer E, Bernard A, et al. Bone marrow CD34+/B220+ progenitors target the inflamed brain and display in vitro differentiation potential toward microglia. FASEB J. 2006;20:2081–92.
54. Chung S, Rho S, Kim G, Kim SR, Baek KH, Kang M. Human umbilical cord blood mononuclear cells and chorionic plate-derived mesenchymal stem cells promote axon survival in a rat model of optic nerve crush injury. Int J Mol Med. 2016;37:1170–80.
55. Touyama M, Touyama J, Toyokawa S, Kobayashi Y. Trends in the prevalence of cerebral palsy in children born between 1988 and 2007 in Okinawa, Japan. Brain Dev. 2016;38:792–9.
56. Koterazawa K, Okada Y, Miyata H. Incidence of cerebral palsy in Himeji over a 25-year period. No Hattatsu. 2016;48:14–9. Japanese
57. Glinianaia SV, Best KE, Lingam R, Rankin J. Predicting the prevalence of cerebral palsy by severity level in children aged 3 to 15 years across England and Wales by 2020. Dev Med Child Neurol. 2017;59(8):864–70.

Chapter 3
Pathophysiology and Pathology of Neonatal Hypoxic-Ischemic Encephalopathy

Masahiro Hayakawa

Abstract Hypoxic-ischemic encephalopathy (HIE) is one of the most important diseases in perinatal medicine. The pathophysiology and pathology of HIE are quite unique. The mode of cell death includes necrosis and apoptosis. Necrosis occurs in conditions of primary energy failure following the initial injury. On the other hand, apoptosis occurs days after the initial injury. The damaged area in the brain depends on the mode of injury. Severe and prolonged insults result in diffuse and marked neuronal necrosis. The cerebral cortex-deep nuclear pattern of neuronal injury appears to be related to insults that are less severe and due to partial asphyxia. The deep nuclear-brainstem pattern of injury to the basal ganglia-thalamus-brainstem occurs in infants with total asphyxia.

Keywords Hypoxic-ischemic encephalopathy · Primary energy failure · Secondary energy failure · Total asphyxia · Partial asphyxia

3.1 Introduction

Hypoxia-ischemia in the perinatal period is an important cause of neurological sequelae and associated disabilities in children. In Japan, the incidence of moderate to severe hypoxic-ischemic encephalopathy (HIE) is reported to be 0.37/1000 births. Infants with moderate to severe HIE tend to develop cerebral palsy (CP) [1]. CP is one of the most costly neurologic disabilities (about 100 million JPY/patient) because of its persistence over the life span. In a term infant, the most common mechanism of hypoxic injury is intrauterine asphyxia brought on by circulatory problems, such as clotting of placental arteries, placental abruption, or

M. Hayakawa, M.D., Ph.D.
Division of Neonatology, Center for Maternal-Neonatal Care,
Nagoya University Hospital, Nagoya, Japan
e-mail: masahaya@med.nagoya-u.ac.jp

© Springer Nature Singapore Pte Ltd. 2018

H. Shintaku et al. (eds.), *Cell Therapy for Perinatal Brain Injury*,
https://doi.org/10.1007/978-981-10-1412-3_3

inflammatory processes. These result in perinatal depression leading to diminished exchange of oxygen and carbon dioxide and severe lactic acidosis. In this chapter, the pathophysiology and pathology of HIE are reviewed.

3.2 The Mode of Cell Death in Hypoxic-Ischemic Encephalopathy

There are two fundamental modes of cell death in the nervous system, necrosis and apoptosis. It is now clear that hypoxic-ischemic insults may lead to necrosis and/or apoptosis, which is dependent principally on the severity of the insult and the maturational state of the cell. Certain characteristics readily distinguish these two forms of cell death. Necrotic cell death is characterized by cytoplasmic vacuolation, membrane disintegration, cell rupture, and release of intracellular contents. As a consequence, inflammation and phagocytosis subsequently occur. By contrast, apoptosis is characterized by condensation and margination of chromatin, cell shrinkage, relative preservation of cellular membranes, and cell death without inflammation.

3.3 The Primary and Secondary Energy Failure in Hypoxic-Ischemic Encephalopathy (Fig. 3.1)

Primary energy failure occurs as a result of the initial reduction of cerebral blood flow [2]. The impairment of cerebral blood flow leads to decreases in oxygen and glucose levels, which lead to significantly less adenosine triphosphate (ATP) and increased lactate production [3]. Low ATP levels cause the failure of many of the mechanisms that maintain cell integrity, particularly the sodium/potassium (Na^+/K^+) pumps and mechanisms to maintain low intracellular calcium. When the Na^+/K^+ pumps fail, an excessive influx of Na^+ precipitates massive depolarization of neurons. This leads to the release of glutamate, a prominent excitatory neurotransmitter. The glutamate binds to AMPA/kainate and NMDA glutamate receptors, allowing additional influx of intracellular calcium and sodium [4]. Increased intracellular calcium has significant detrimental effects, which lead to cerebral edema, ischemia, and microvascular damage, with resultant necrosis and/or apoptosis. Most of the effects of primary energy failure lead to cellular necrosis through impaired cellular integrity and disruption of the cytoskeleton and cell membrane.

Necrosis occurs in conditions of very severe hypoxia and ischemia [4]. This causes cells to swell and rupture, leading to cell death. Upon rupture, cellular contents are released, leading to inflammation. When inflammation occurs, there is an influx of microglia to the area, which release inflammatory mediators [5]. Inflammatory mediators can damage the white matter and lead to formation of scar tissue. If the insult is less severe, the cells may recover or progress to apoptosis [4].

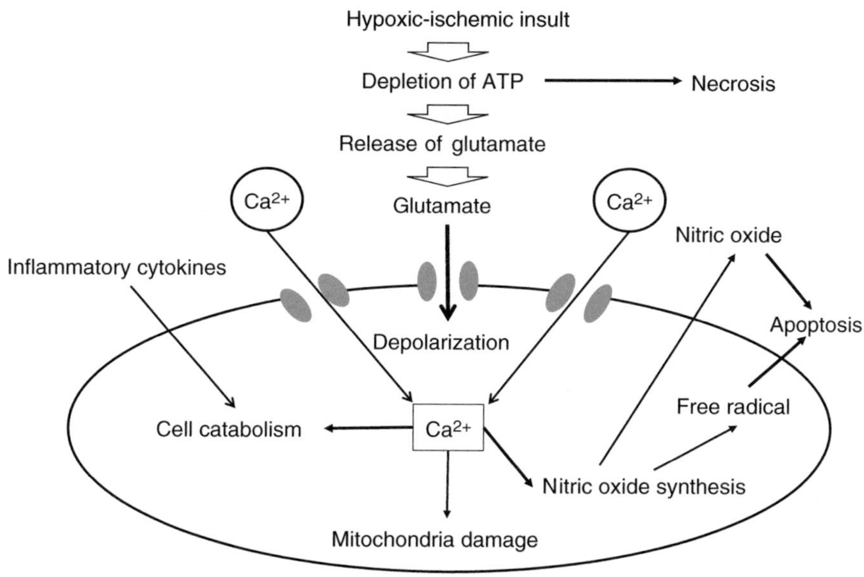

Fig. 3.1 Cell death pathway involved in hypoxic-ischemic brain injury

Apoptosis causes cell shrinkage and general preservation of the cellular membranes with no associated inflammation. Apoptosis can occur days following the initial injury [6]. Both necrosis and apoptosis can lead to decreased brain function.

The extent of primary energy failure contributes to further injury during the secondary energy failure phase. If the hypoxic-ischemic insult is severe, neuronal cell death can occur through necrosis [5]. Once blood flow is restored, there is a brief period of recovery. This brief recovery is the latent period, which is characterized by normal cerebral metabolism. The latent period is thought to vary depending on the extent and severity of the hypoxic-ischemic insult; the more severe the insult, the shorter the latent period is [7]. Currently, the exact timing of the primary energy failure phase, the latent period, and the beginning and ending of the secondary energy failure phase remain unknown [8]. The latent period is considered the optimal timing for therapeutic interventions.

The secondary energy failure phase occurs 6–48 h after the initial injury. The exact mechanisms of secondary energy failure remain unclear but appear to be related to oxidative stress, excitotoxicity, and inflammation. The overproduction of free radicals, which cause damage to neuronal cell membranes and lead to necrosis or apoptosis, causes oxidative stress. Oxidative stress is particularly harmful to the neonatal brain [9] due to low concentrations of antioxidants and a high consumption of oxygen when transitioning from the fetal to neonatal life [10]. Neonates also have high concentrations of unsaturated fatty acids that break down to form more oxygen free radicals. During a hypoxic-ischemic state, protein-bound iron is released, which makes Fe^{2+} available to react with peroxides and form free radicals. The increased susceptibility to free radical formation and the decreased ability of the neonatal brain to eliminate free radicals lead to damage of neuronal tissue. Excitotoxicity occurs when excessive levels of extracellular neurotransmitters, especially glutamate, overstimulate excitatory receptors. The overstimulation allows additional influx of sodium and calcium into neural cells. Glutamate is used by a variety of neuronal pathways, including hearing, vision, somatosensory function, and learning and memory, which can account for the disruptive effect of HIE on subsequent development. Inflammation is also thought to be important in the development of the HIE-related brain injury [10].

3.4 Pathophysiology of Hypoxic-Ischemic Encephalopathy in a Term Neonate (Fig. 3.2)

A reduction of oxygenation to the fetus leads to bradycardia, which reduces cerebral perfusion pressure as well as oxygenation of neural tissue. The degree to which oxygenation is impaired can also vary. The extent of damage will depend on the degree of impaired oxygenation and the duration of impaired oxygenation; the more severe the degree of impaired oxygenation and the longer the duration of impaired oxygenation, the greater the risk of permanent neurological injury. Additionally, the rapidity of onset of the decrease in flow influences the pattern of injury seen in the brain. In such situations, the fetus faces a sudden profound asphyxia, often termed total asphyxia [11], with a marginally less severe asphyxia which is referred to as near-total asphyxia. This event represents a complete interruption in the supply of oxygen. This total lack of oxygen can be tolerated for only a relatively brief period of time before there is permanent neurological damage and can potentially lead to fetal death. With a sudden decrease in blood flow and oxygen, there is little time for the redistribution of blood flow to protect more mature neurons in the central gray matter of the basal ganglia, thalamus, and brainstem. The relative maturity or immaturity of the developing brain increases or decreases the vulnerability of the tissues to the effects of a decrease in oxygenation and blood flow. Neurons that are mature

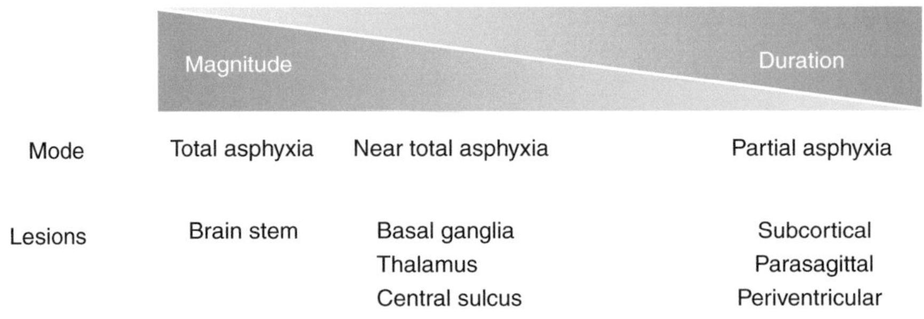

Fig. 3.2 The relationship between mode of injury and lesions

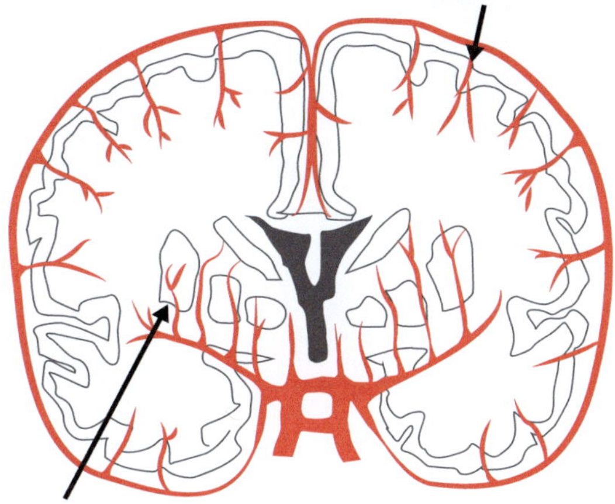

Fig. 3.3 Anatomical characteristics of arteries in cortex/subcortex/white matter

and functional are more vulnerable to a lack of nutrients, whereas cortical areas of the brain that are immature and nonfunctional are accustomed to the relatively hypoxic in utero environment and are less vulnerable [12].

Where the degree of impaired oxygen delivery is less dramatic, the fetus faces partial asphyxia. The fetus is equipped with a number of compensatory strategies that allow it to withstand impaired oxygen gas exchange for hours. The ultimate impact of impaired gas exchange on the fetus will depend on the duration and magnitude of the insult. With a more gradual onset of decreased flow and oxygen, there is time for a relative shift of flow to protect more valuable and vulnerable structures. With a shift in blood flow to the brainstem and central gray matter, the burden of the injury falls on the supratentorial distal portions of the cortex and white matter, in the so-called watershed zones located between the vascular territories (Fig. 3.3), between the anterior and middle cerebral arteries, and between the posterior and middle cerebral arteries (Figs. 3.4 and 3.5).

A fetus may suffer from a partial asphyxia, which is then followed by a total asphyxia. In these circumstances, the fetus is said to have suffered from a "mixed pattern" of asphyxia.

3.4.1 Near-Total Asphyxia

A sudden, marked, or catastrophic decrease in cerebral blood flow or oxygenation to the fetal brain or newborn infant produces near-total asphyxia [11]. The three most common causes for this decrease are placental abruption, cord prolapse, and uterine rupture [13]. Most near-total asphyxia cases are terminal events occurring immediately before delivery. Near-total asphyxia can also occur in a fetus in utero

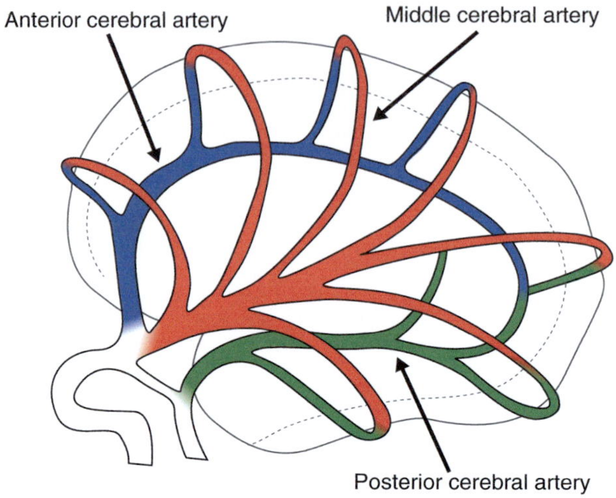

Fig. 3.4 Anatomical characteristics of the three major cerebral arteries

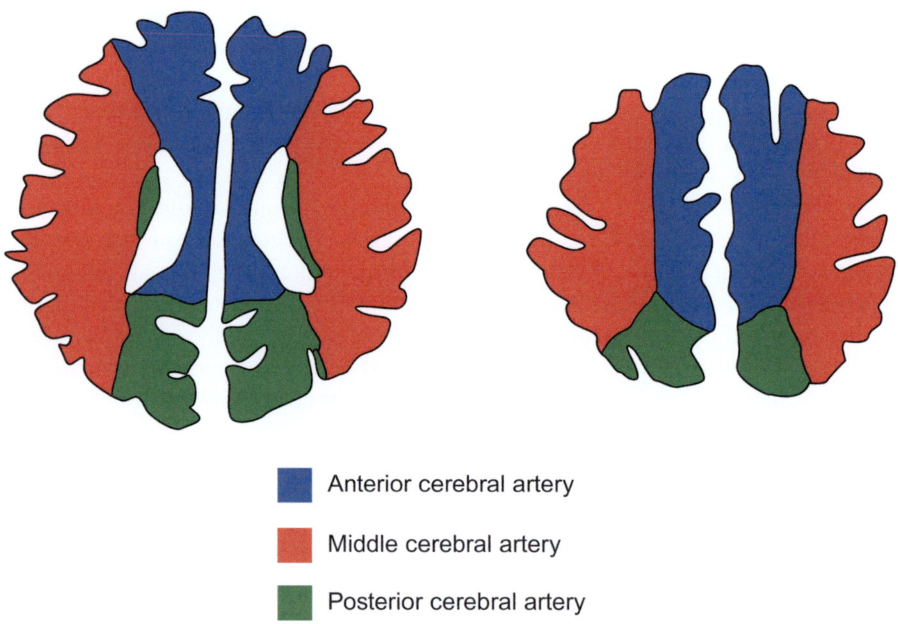

Fig. 3.5 Territories of the major three cerebral arteries

before labor and delivery when the mother experiences a cardiac arrest or cardiovascular collapse as the result of a reaction to an anesthetic or other drugs, has a vasovagal reaction, or goes into shock secondary to trauma, for example, in a motor vehicle accident.

Vulnerability to near-total asphyxia in a term infant is manifested in mature neurons with high metabolic rates that are most sensitive to the deprivation of nutrients [14]. Such regions of vulnerability include the posterior putamina, ventrolateral nucleus of the thalamus, pre- and postcentral gyri (the rolandic cortex region that lies along the central sulcus), and subrolandic white matter that is an area of active myelination at term [12]. In addition, the hippocampi, the superior vermis, and multiple small areas within the brainstem, primarily the cranial nerve nuclei and internal capsules, are also highly sensitive to profound asphyxia [15]. More extensive areas of the basal ganglia can be involved, including other portions of the thalami, the full putamina, globus pallidus, and caudate nuclei. Extensive injuries to the basal ganglia are less common than injuries to the putamen.

3.4.2 Partial Asphyxia

As the fetus comes to full term, the watershed zones in the brain, the areas between vascular territories, shift from the periventricular region toward the cortex and the subcortical white matter (Fig. 3.3). The watershed regions lie anteriorly between the anterior and middle cerebral arteries, primarily in the parasagittal region of the anterior frontal and parietal lobes, and posteriorly between the middle and posterior cerebral arteries in the parasagittal region of the posterior parietal and occipital lobes (Fig. 3.5). There is also an inferior watershed zone in the region of the posterior inferior temporal lobes. Additionally, there is a watershed region between the branches of the vertebral and basilar arteries between the superior cerebellar, posterior inferior cerebellar, and anterior cerebellar arteries in the cerebellum; however, this watershed is rarely found to be involved in a term infant with hypoxic-ischemic brain injury. Watershed territory injuries of the supratentorial brain occur in term fetuses and neonates when there is a reduction in blood flow and oxygenation. The partial asphyxic pattern of injury may occur silently in utero during the last weeks of gestation and become manifest following delivery or at a later point in time. More often it is recognized during the labor and delivery period, when it is associated with events such as cord compression with a nuchal cord, oligohydramnios producing cord compression, or placental insufficiency owing to abnormalities of placental growth and development. Such injuries are most frequently gradual in onset, leading to a progressive but significant reduction in blood flow and oxygenation to the tissue at the end of the vessels in the watershed zones [16]. A series of such events occurring over 1 or more hours results in variable injury to either or both the gray and white matter at the site of the watershed zone. Prolongation of the insult can produce involvement extending beyond the usual watershed region and involving greater portions of the cerebral hemispheres. With further depletion of energy reserves and further diminishing of the fetal heart rate, a pattern of injury may develop that has elements of a partial and near-total asphyxia.

In severe partial asphyxia, the period of reduced blood flow and oxygenation goes on for a sufficiently long time or to a sufficient degree of deprivation of nutrients that the area of cerebral cortical gray matter and subcortical white matter involvement extends beyond the typical watershed areas of the brain. This involvement produces a more homogeneous and extensive pattern of cortical and subcortical injury with edema and resultant mass effects that tend to involve large portions or all of the cerebral lobes bilaterally.

3.4.3 *Mixed Partial Prolonged Asphyxia Leading to Terminal Profound Asphyxia*

A mixed form of asphyxic injury occurs when energy substrates are depleted in partial asphyxia, leading to a further insult in the form of a terminal near-total collapse. This injury is seen clinically as a sudden bradycardic event superimposed on a prior more gradual abnormal decline in fetal heart rate. In addition to the damage from the partial asphyxia occurring in, or beyond, the watershed regions, the addition of severe bradycardic events causes injury to the thalamus and putamina with the possibility of hippocampal, vermian, and brainstem injury as well.

3.5 Pathology of Hypoxic-Ischemic Encephalopathy

3.5.1 *Selective Neuronal Necrosis*

Selective neuronal necrosis is the most common injury response observed after intrapartum hypoxic ischemia. The patterns include diffuse neuronal injury, cerebral cortex-deep nuclear neuronal injury, and deep nuclear-brainstem neuronal injury.

Excitotoxicity is believed to be responsible for the neuronal damage caused by hypoxic ischemia in the developing brain [17]. There is evidence that the neuronal pattern of damage reflects the dysfunction of a set of excitatory neuronal circuits triggering selective neuronal death [18]. Brain injury after transient hypoxic ischemia is an evolving process; transient severe hypoxic ischemia and subsequent reperfusion/reoxygenation lead not only to immediate cell death but trigger complex biochemical events, which result in further delayed neuronal death [19]. However, apoptotic cell death is currently considered to be the main cause of delayed neuronal death based on evidence from hypoxic ischemia in animal models and human infants who subsequently died.

Factors related to the severity and the temporal characteristics of the insult appear to be of particular importance in determining the major pattern of selective neuronal injury in the newborn. Diffuse neuronal injury typically occurs following a very severe, very prolonged insult. The major sites which typically develop diffuse neuronal necrosis in a term infant include the cerebral cortex, hippocampus, deep nuclear structures (the caudate, putamen, and thalamus), and brainstem.

Cerebral-deep nuclear neuronal injury usually occurs following a moderate to severe, prolonged insult and typically consists of injury to the perirolandic cortex/putamen and thalamus. Deep nuclear-brainstem neuronal injury typically follows a severe, abrupt insult. The brainstem, thalamus, and basal ganglia have an active metabolism, and corresponding blood flow is abundant in these areas making them most vulnerable to acute anoxia.

It is postulated that adaptive mechanisms normally operate during asphyxic events. In the most profound and severe insults, blood diverts from the cerebral hemisphere to vital deep nuclear structures. Since deep nuclear structures have high rates of energy use, these nuclei are particularly likely to be injured. In the most prolonged and less severe insults, the diversion of blood to deep nuclear structures occurs, at least to a degree, and the cerebral regions are more likely to be injured after brief, repeated hypoxic-ischemic insults [20, 21].

3.5.2 *Parasagittal Cerebral Injury*

Parasagittal cerebral injury is a lesion of the cerebral cortex and subcortical white matter with a characteristic distribution over the superomedial aspects of the cerebral convexities [22]. This pattern of injury is characterized by necrosis of the cortex and the immediately adjacent white matter and usually affects the parieto-occipital regions (the posterior watershed) more than the anterior watershed. The precuneus is an area of the brain that lies at the junction of all three major cerebral arteries and is particularly vulnerable to damage in this pattern of injury. At the cellular level, laminar necrosis of cortical pyramidal neurons is typically seen. The likely areas of greatest ischemia relate to parasagittal vascular anatomical factors. Thus, the areas of necrosis in parasagittal cerebral injury are in the border zones between the end fields of the major cerebral arteries (Figs. 3.4 and 3.5). These border zones are the brain regions most susceptible to a fall in cerebral perfusion pressure. The watershed concept is analogous to an irrigation system supplying a series of fields with water and emphasizes the vulnerability of the last fields when the head of pressure falls.

3.6 Conclusion

HIE is one of the most serious birth complications. The hypoxic-ischemic event can be caused by multiple events, but ultimately brain injury occurs because of impaired cerebral blood flow and oxygen delivery to the brain. The phases of injury are categorized as primary and secondary energy failure with the latent period between the phases being the optimal timing for interventions. The majority of treatment strategies target ameliorating the effects of the secondary energy failure. Nowadays, research for new treatments using stem cells against HIE have been conducted.

However, most of them are basic research using model animals. There are a few clinical trials of stem cell therapies against HIE. We must continue to search for ways to prevent and treat the effects of the hypoxic-ischemic event to improve neurological outcomes in infants with HIE.

References

1. Hayakawa M, Ito Y, Saito S, Mitsuda N, Hosono S, Yoda H, et al. Incidence and prediction of outcome in hypoxic-ischemic encephalopathy in Japan. Pediatr Int. 2014;56(2):215–21. https://doi.org/10.1111/ped.12233.
2. Shalak L, Perlman JM. Hypoxic-ischemic brain injury in the term infant-current concepts. Early Hum Dev. 2004;80(2):125–41. https://doi.org/10.1016/j.earlhumdev.2004.06.003.
3. Hanrahan JD, Sargentoni J, Azzopardi D, Manji K, Cowan FM, Rutherford MA, et al. Cerebral metabolism within 18 hours of birth asphyxia: a proton magnetic resonance spectroscopy study. Pediatr Res. 1996;39(4 Pt 1):584–90. https://doi.org/10.1203/00006450-199604000-00004.
4. Johnston MV, Ishida A, Ishida WN, Matsushita HB, Nishimura A, Tsuji M. Plasticity and injury in the developing brain. Brain and Development. 2009;31(1):1–10. https://doi.org/10.1016/j.braindev.2008.03.014.
5. Alvarez-Diaz A, Hilario E, de Cerio FG, Valls-i-Soler A, Alvarez-Diaz FJ. Hypoxic-ischemic injury in the immature brain--key vascular and cellular players. Neonatology. 2007;92(4):227–35. https://doi.org/10.1159/000103741.
6. Fatemi A, Wilson MA, Johnston MV. Hypoxic-ischemic encephalopathy in the term infant. Clin Perinatol. 2009;36(4):835–858., vii. https://doi.org/10.1016/j.clp.2009.07.011.
7. Iwata O, Iwata S, Thornton JS, De Vita E, Bainbridge A, Herbert L, et al. "Therapeutic time window" duration decreases with increasing severity of cerebral hypoxia-ischaemia under normothermia and delayed hypothermia in newborn piglets. Brain Res. 2007;1154:173–80. https://doi.org/10.1016/j.brainres.2007.03.083.
8. Laptook AR. Use of therapeutic hypothermia for term infants with hypoxic-ischemic encephalopathy. Pediatr Clin North Am. 2009;56(3):601–16. https://doi.org/10.1016/j.pcl.2009.03.007.
9. Buonocore G, Groenendaal F. Anti-oxidant strategies. Semin Fetal Neonatal Med. 2007;12(4):287–95. https://doi.org/10.1016/j.siny.2007.01.020.
10. Ferriero DM. Neonatal brain injury. N Engl J Med. 2004;351(19):1985–95. https://doi.org/10.1056/NEJMra041996.
11. Menkes JH, Curran J. Clinical and MR correlates in children with extrapyramidal cerebral palsy. AJNR Am J Neuroradiol. 1994;15(3):451–7.
12. Counsell SJ, Helber A, Mader I, Staudt M, Wolff M, Groenendaal F, et al. Bilateral lesions of thalamus and basal ganglia: origin and outcome. Dev Med Child Neurol. 2002;44(7):477–84.
13. Leung AS, Leung EK, Paul RH. Uterine rupture after previous cesarean delivery: maternal and fetal consequences. Am J Obstet Gynecol. 1993;169(4):945–50.
14. Pasternak JF, Gorey MT. The syndrome of acute near-total intrauterine asphyxia in the term infant. Pediatr Neurol. 1998;18(5):391–8.
15. Rutherford MA, Pennock JM, Counsell SJ, Mercuri E, Cowan FM, Dubowitz LM, et al. Abnormal magnetic resonance signal in the internal capsule predicts poor neurodevelopmental outcome in infants with hypoxic-ischemic encephalopathy. Pediatrics. 1998;102(2 Pt 1):323–8.
16. De Haan HH, Gunn AJ, Williams CE, Gluckman PD. Brief repeated umbilical cord occlusions cause sustained cytotoxic cerebral edema and focal infarcts in near-term fetal lambs. Pediatr Res. 1997;41(1):96–104. https://doi.org/10.1203/00006450-199704001-00584.
17. Johnston MV, Trescher WH, Ishida A, Nakajima W. Neurobiology of hypoxic-ischemic injury in the developing brain. Pediatr Res. 2001;49(6):735–41. https://doi.org/10.1203/00006450-200106000-00003.

18. McDonald JW, Johnston MV. Physiological and pathophysiological roles of excitatory amino acids during central nervous system development. Brain Res Brain Res Rev. 1990;15(1):41–70.
19. Orrenius S, Zhivotovsky B, Nicotera P. Regulation of cell death: the calcium-apoptosis link. Nat Rev Mol Cell Biol. 2003;4(7):552–65. https://doi.org/10.1038/nrm1150.
20. Mallard EC, Waldvogel HJ, Williams CE, Faull RL, Gluckman PD. Repeated asphyxia causes loss of striatal projection neurons in the fetal sheep brain. Neuroscience. 1995;65(3):827–36.
21. Mallard EC, Williams CE, Johnston BM, Gunning MI, Davis S, Gluckman PD. Repeated episodes of umbilical cord occlusion in fetal sheep lead to preferential damage to the striatum and sensitize the heart to further insults. Pediatr Res. 1995;37(6):707–13. https://doi.org/10.1203/00006450-199506000-00006.
22. Sato Y, Hayakawa M, Iwata O, Okumura A, Kato T, Hayakawa F, et al. Delayed neurological signs following isolated parasagittal injury in asphyxia at term. Eur J Paediatr Neurol. 2008;12(5):359–65. https://doi.org/10.1016/j.ejpn.2007.10.003.

Chapter 4
Neural Stem/Progenitor Cells for Perinatal Brain Injury

Yoshiaki Sato

Abstract Cell transplantation therapy is a potential treatment for neonatal brain injury. Neural stem/progenitor cells (NSPCs) are defined as cells that have abilities for self-renewal and differentiation into neurons, astrocytes, and oligodendrocytes. There are several origins of NSPCs, namely, ES cell-derived NSPCs, iPS-derived NSPCs, fetal NSPCs, and adult NSPCs.

NSPCs were formerly the cell type most commonly studied in the early period in the stem cell research to develop novel therapies for neuronal diseases. There are several experimental studies using NSPCs for the treatment of perinatal brain injuries. However, there has been only one clinical trial using NSPCs for neonatal brain injury to date. In the clinical application of NSPC treatment for neonatal brain injury, we would encounter greater difficulty due to ethical considerations when preparing the cells. In addition, we must consider the invasive approach for injection of cells.

In this chapter, I describe the various origins of NSPCs as well as preclinical and clinical studies involving NSPCs.

Keywords Neural stem/progenitor cells · Neural lineage · Neuron · Astrocyte · Oligodendrocyte

4.1 Introduction

Stem cells are derived from various tissues and are defined by their properties of self-renewal and multipotency. They are capable of generating committed progenitor cells to variable degrees and ultimately differentiating into mature cells. Cell transplantation therapy is a potential treatment for neonatal brain injury. So far,

Y. Sato, M.D., Ph.D.
Division of Neonatology, Center for Maternal-Neonatal Care, Nagoya University Hospital, Nagoya, Japan
e-mail: yoshiaki@med.nagoya-u.ac.jp

© Springer Nature Singapore Pte Ltd. 2018
H. Shintaku et al. (eds.), *Cell Therapy for Perinatal Brain Injury*,
https://doi.org/10.1007/978-981-10-1412-3_4

several kinds of stem cells have been investigated as "a player" in cell transplantation therapy including embryonic stem (ES) cells, neural stem/progenitor cells (NSPCs), bone marrow stromal cells, umbilical cord stem cells, and induced pluripotent stem (iPS) cells [1].

NSPCs are defined as cells that have abilities for self-renewal and differentiation into neurons, astrocytes, and oligodendrocytes. Their differentiated cell types depend on the stage of development and the region from which they are isolated [2–4], and the proliferation and differentiation of NSPCs are regulated by both intrinsic factors, such as transcription factors, and extrinsic factors, such as growth factors including fibroblast growth factors (FGFs) and epidermal growth factors (EGFs) [5].

In this chapter, I describe the various origins of NSPCs as well as preclinical and clinical studies involving NSPCs.

4.2 Origins of NSPCs

There are several origins of NSPCs that have been studied, namely, ES cell-derived NSPCs, iPS-derived NSPCs, fetal NSPCs, and adult NSPCs.

ES cells are pluripotent cells isolated from the inner cell mass of blastocysts. ES cells have an indefinite self-renewal capacity as well as an ability to differentiate into all cell types derived from the three embryonic germ layers [6, 7]. The proliferation and pluripotent capacities of ES cells are the highest of all stem cell types; however, the high degree of pluripotency could easily lead to teratoma formation [1]. Therefore, it is necessary to restrict ES cells to a neuronal lineage for cell transplantation therapy. Many research groups have strived to establish methods to generate a highly enriched population of NSPCs from ES cells, and two major methods have since been developed: exposure of ES cells to retinoic acid [8–10] and selection of NSPCs from cultures of ES cells in the presence of FGF-2 [11]. Several selective markers have been found for NSPCs including nestin, Lewis X, PNA, HSA, Musashi-1, and Sox1. Ethical constraints are a potential problem for the use of ES cells for transplantation therapy. There are still very few countries that have clear legislation for the usage of human blastocysts.

Pluripotent cells were originally induced from differentiated cells such as skin fibroblasts [12]. These induced cells (iPS cells) exhibit morphology and growth properties similar to those of ES cells and express ES cell marker genes. Since iPS cells can be established from the cells of individual patients, they can generate autologous NSPCs for transplantation. Although the tumorigenicity of these cells must be overcome, as in the case of ES cells, they are promising as a source of stem cells for transplantation therapy in the future.

Fetal NSPCs are directly isolated from embryonic or fetal brains and usually propagated in culture as neurospheres in the presence of EGF and FGF-2 [13]. Adult NSPCs persist in the subventricular zone and the hippocampal subgranular zone throughout life [14–16] and can be also isolated from these areas and propagated in the same way as fetal NSPCs [17, 18]. Since NSPCs are more lineage-restricted than ES cells, they have a lower possibility to form tumors after transplantation. Ethical considerations need to be addressed prior to the use of postmortem human brains as a source of NSPCs in future clinical applications. In addition, the limited availability is a potential disadvantage for adult NSPCs; however, adult NSPCs have a potential advantage, namely, a possibility to generate autologous transplantation of cells prepared from small biopsies of neural tissues from patients themselves.

4.3 Preclinical Studies for Perinatal Brain Injury with NSPCs

NSPCs were formerly the cell type most commonly studied in the early period in the stem cell research to develop novel therapies for neuronal diseases. There are several experimental studies using NSPCs for the treatment of perinatal brain injuries.

First, Park et al. in 2002 [19], showed that seeding NSPCs onto a polymer scaffold that was subsequently implanted into the hypoxic-ischemic infarction cavities dramatically reduced parenchymal loss. These authors also showed the effect of hypoxia-ischemia (HI) on the migration and differentiation of NSPCs [20] and that neurotrophin-3-expressing NSPCs could increase the rate of neuronal differentiation from 5 to >80% [21]. Imitola et al. demonstrated the inflammatory mechanisms involved in the migration of NSPCs in HI [22]. Mueller et al. transplanted human embryonic germ cell-derived neural stem cells into the forebrain of neonatal mice with excitotoxic brain damage and showed that these cells differentiated into neuronal and glial cells and replace lost neurons [23].

Our group evaluated a strategy for the treatment of perinatal brain injury using a combination of neural cell/tissue transplantation with niche modification [1]. Chondroitin sulfate proteoglycans (CSPGs) are one of the major components of the extracellular matrix in the central nervous system (CNS) and are involved in various cellular events in the formation and maintenance of the neural network [24]. Chondroitinase ABC (ChABC) treatment, which degrades glycosaminoglycan (GAG) side chains of CSPGs, combined with NSPC grafts has been shown to promote the migration of grafted NSPCs and axonal regeneration after injury of the mature spinal cord. In addition, CSPGs in the substrata impair neural cell attachment, and removal of chondroitin sulfate (CS) by ChABC digestion can intensify cell attachment to the substratum [1]. Injection of NSPCs with ChABC into the injured neonatal brain may help the adhesion and/or migration of NSPCs to the injured site and may reduce neuronal brain injury. In our study, intracerebroventricular injection of NSPCs with ChABC, not NSPCs alone, reduced brain injury in a rat neonatal HI model [25].

Subsequently, several publications with neural stem cells for perinatal brain injury emerged. Comi et al. used postnatal day 12 CD1 mice with right-sided carotid ligation. Two or 7 days after ligation, mice received an intrastriatal injection of B5 ES cell-derived neural stem cells. Pups receiving stem cells 2 days but not 7 days after ligation had less severe hemispheric brain atrophy [26]. Daadi et al. showed that human neural stem cell derived from human ES cells transplanted into the forebrain 24 h after the induction of HI significantly improved the use of the contralateral impeded forelimb in the rotarod test and upregulated genes involved in neurogenesis, gliogenesis, and neurotrophic support when examined with microarray analysis [27]. Zheng et al. revealed that with VEGF transfection, NSPCs were marginally better than when they had not been transfected [28]. Shinoyama et al. injected mice embryonic stem cell-derived NSPCs into the deep layer of the motor cortex in the HI brain, and ES-NPCs could differentiate to cortical neurons with pyramidal morphology, and the motor functions of the transplanted HI mice also improved significantly [29]. Wang et al. evaluated the combination therapy with mild hypothermia. The neuroprotective effects of mild hypothermia combined with neural stem cell transplantation are superior to those of monotherapy [30]. Furthermore, Ashwal et al. demonstrated that the treatment effects of neural stem cells in neonatal rats with HI injury are not influenced by host gender [31]. Hsueh et al. differentiated adipose-derived stem cells (ASCs) toward the progenitor of endothelial progenitor cells (EPCs) and neural precursor cells (NPCs) and showed the synergy of these cells allowed improvements in cognitive and motor functions [32].

4.4 Clinical Studies for Perinatal Brain Injury Using NSPCs

According to ClinicalTrials.gov (https://clinicaltrials.gov/), there has been only one clinical trial using NSPCs for neonatal brain injury to date. This is an ongoing study performed by Luna et al. in the Navy General Hospital, Beijing, China (NCT02854579), to investigate the efficacy and safety of allogenic NSPCs, derived from the aborted human fetal forebrain, as well as paracrine factors of human mesenchymal stem cells for patients with moderate/severe hypoxic-ischemic encephalopathy (HIE). In this study, patients with HIE received (will receive) intrathecal injection of NSPCs, or concentrated paracrine factors of human mesenchymal stem cells, both, or no intervention. This group has already shown the efficacy of NSPC transplantation into the lateral ventricle in children with severe cerebral palsy [33].

Although there are several preclinical studies (as shown in the previous section), we would encounter greater difficulty in the clinical application of NSPC treatment for neonatal brain injury due to ethical considerations when preparing the cells (described in the second section). In addition, we must consider the invasive approach for injection of cells as intracerebral injection was used in all preclinical studies.

4.5 Conclusions

In this chapter, the various origins of NSPCs and preclinical and clinical studies with NSPCs for perinatal HI were reviewed. NSPCs were widely studied in the early period for neuronal diseases, and there are several preclinical studies for perinatal HI. However, due to ethical considerations when preparing the cells as well as the invasive approach for injection of cells, the clinical application using NSPCs for perinatal HI is still challenging.

References

1. Sato Y, Oohira A. Chondroitin sulfate, a major niche substance of neural stem cells, and cell transplantation therapy of neurodegeneration combined with niche modification. Curr Stem Cell Res Ther. 2009;4(3):200–9.
2. Hack MA, Sugimori M, Lundberg C, Nakafuku M, Gotz M. Regionalization and fate specification in neurospheres: the role of Olig2 and Pax6. Mol Cell Neurosci. 2004;25(4):664–78. https://doi.org/10.1016/j.mcn.2003.12.012[doi]S1044743103003956[pii].
3. Horiguchi S, Takahashi J, Kishi Y, Morizane A, Okamoto Y, Koyanagi M, et al. Neural precursor cells derived from human embryonic brain retain regional specificity. J Neurosci Res. 2004;75(6):817–24. https://doi.org/10.1002/jnr.20046.
4. Nery S, Fishell G, Corbin JG. The caudal ganglionic eminence is a source of distinct cortical and subcortical cell populations. Nat Neurosci. 2002;5(12):1279–87. https://doi.org/10.1038/nn971[doi]nn971[pii].
5. Alvarez-Buylla A, Lim DA. For the long run: maintaining germinal niches in the adult brain. Neuron. 2004;41(5):683–6.
6. Evans MJ, Kaufman MH. Establishment in culture of pluripotential cells from mouse embryos. Nature. 1981;292(5819):154–6.
7. Martin GR. Isolation of a pluripotent cell line from early mouse embryos cultured in medium conditioned by teratocarcinoma stem cells. Proc Natl Acad Sci U S A. 1981;78(12):7634–8.
8. Bain G, Kitchens D, Yao M, Huettner JE, Gottlieb DI. Embryonic stem cells express neuronal properties in vitro. Dev Biol. 1995;168(2):342–57. https://doi.org/10.1006/dbio.1995.1085.
9. Fraichard A, Chassande O, Bilbaut G, Dehay C, Savatier P, Samarut J. In vitro differentiation of embryonic stem cells into glial cells and functional neurons. J Cell Sci. 1995;108(Pt 10):3181–8.
10. Strubing C, Ahnert-Hilger G, Shan J, Wiedenmann B, Hescheler J, Wobus AM. Differentiation of pluripotent embryonic stem cells into the neuronal lineage in vitro gives rise to mature inhibitory and excitatory neurons. Mech Dev. 1995;53(2):275–87. https://doi.org/10.1016/0925-4773(95)00446-8.
11. Okabe S, Forsberg-Nilsson K, Spiro AC, Segal M, McKay RD. Development of neuronal precursor cells and functional postmitotic neurons from embryonic stem cells in vitro. Mech Dev. 1996;59(1):89–102. https://doi.org/10.1016/0925-4773(96)00572-2.
12. Takahashi K, Yamanaka S. Induction of pluripotent stem cells from mouse embryonic and adult fibroblast cultures by defined factors. Cell. 2006;126:663–76.
13. Johe KK, Hazel TG, Muller T, Dugich-Djordjevic MM, McKay RD. Single factors direct the differentiation of stem cells from the fetal and adult central nervous system. Genes Dev. 1996;10(24):3129–40.
14. Eriksson PS, Perfilieva E, Bjork-Eriksson T, Alborn AM, Nordborg C, Peterson DA, et al. Neurogenesis in the adult human hippocampus. Nat Med. 1998;4:1313–7.

15. Gould E, Beylin A, Tanapat P, Reeves A, Shors TJ. Learning enhances adult neurogenesis in the hippocampal formation. Nat Neurosci. 1999;2:260–5.
16. Luskin MB. Restricted proliferation and migration of postnatally generated neurons derived from the forebrain subventricular zone. Neuron. 1993;11:173–89.
17. Morshead CM, Reynolds BA, Craig CG, McBurney MW, Staines WA, Morassutti D, et al. Neural stem cells in the adult mammalian forebrain: a relatively quiescent subpopulation of subependymal cells. Neuron. 1994;13(5):1071–82. https://doi.org/10.1016/0896-6273(94)90046-9.
18. Roy NS, Wang S, Jiang L, Kang J, Benraiss A, Harrison-Restelli C, et al. In vitro neurogenesis by progenitor cells isolated from the adult human hippocampus. Nat Med. 2000;6(3):271–7. https://doi.org/10.1038/73119.
19. Park KI, Teng YD, Snyder EY. The injured brain interacts reciprocally with neural stem cells supported by scaffolds to reconstitute lost tissue. Nat Biotechnol. 2002;20(11):1111–7. https://doi.org/10.1038/nbt751.
20. Park KI, Hack MA, Ourednik J, Yandava B, Flax JD, Stieg PE, et al. Acute injury directs the migration, proliferation, and differentiation of solid organ stem cells: evidence from the effect of hypoxia-ischemia in the CNS on clonal "reporter" neural stem cells. Exp Neurol. 2006a;199(1):156–78. https://doi.org/10.1016/j.expneurol.2006.04.002.
21. Park KI, Himes BT, Stieg PE, Tessler A, Fischer I, Snyder EY. Neural stem cells may be uniquely suited for combined gene therapy and cell replacement: evidence from engraftment of Neurotrophin-3-expressing stem cells in hypoxic-ischemic brain injury. Exp Neurol. 2006b;199(1):179–90. https://doi.org/10.1016/j.expneurol.2006.03.016.
22. Imitola J, Raddassi K, Park KI, Mueller FJ, Nieto M, Teng YD, et al. Directed migration of neural stem cells to sites of CNS injury by the stromal cell-derived factor 1alpha/CXC chemokine receptor 4 pathway. Proc Natl Acad Sci U S A. 2004;101(52):18117–22. https://doi.org/10.1073/pnas.0408258102.
23. Mueller D, Shamblott MJ, Fox HE, Gearhart JD, Martin LJ. Transplanted human embryonic germ cell-derived neural stem cells replace neurons and oligodendrocytes in the forebrain of neonatal mice with excitotoxic brain damage. J Neurosci Res. 2005;82(5):592–608. https://doi.org/10.1002/jnr.20673.
24. Oohira A, Matsui F, Tokita Y, Yamauchi S, Aono S. Molecular interactions of neural chondroitin sulfate proteoglycans in the brain development. Arch Biochem Biophys. 2000;374(1):24–34. https://doi.org/10.1006/abbi.1999.1598.
25. Sato Y, Nakanishi K, Hayakawa M, Kakizawa H, Saito A, Kuroda Y, et al. Reduction of brain injury in neonatal hypoxic-ischemic rats by intracerebroventricular injection of neural stem/progenitor cells together with chondroitinase ABC. Reprod Sci. 2008;15(6):613–20. https://doi.org/10.1177/1933719108317299.
26. Comi AM, Cho E, Mulholland JD, Hooper A, Li Q, Qu Y, et al. Neural stem cells reduce brain injury after unilateral carotid ligation. Pediatric Neurol. 2008;38(2):86–92. https://doi.org/10.1016/j.pediatrneurol.2007.10.007.
27. Daadi MM, Davis AS, Arac A, Li Z, Maag AL, Bhatnagar R, et al. Human neural stem cell grafts modify microglial response and enhance axonal sprouting in neonatal hypoxic-ischemic brain injury. Stroke. 2010;41(3):516–23. https://doi.org/10.1161/strokeaha.109.573691.
28. Zheng XR, Zhang SS, Yin F, Tang JL, Yang YJ, Wang X, et al. Neuroprotection of VEGF-expression neural stem cells in neonatal cerebral palsy rats. Behav Brain Res. 2012;230(1):108–15. https://doi.org/10.1016/j.bbr.2012.01.026.
29. Shinoyama M, Ideguchi M, Kida H, Kajiwara K, Kagawa Y, Maeda Y, et al. Cortical region-specific engraftment of embryonic stem cell-derived neural progenitor cells restores axonal sprouting to a subcortical target and achieves motor functional recovery in a mouse model of neonatal hypoxic-ischemic brain injury. Front Cell Neurosci. 2013;7:128. https://doi.org/10.3389/fncel.2013.00128.
30. Wang L, Jiang F, Li Q, He X, Ma J. Mild hypothermia combined with neural stem cell transplantation for hypoxic-ischemic encephalopathy: neuroprotective effects of combined therapy. Neural Regen Res. 2014;9(19):1745–52. https://doi.org/10.4103/1673-5374.143417.

31. Ashwal S, Ghosh N, Turenius CI, Dulcich M, Denham CM, Tone B, et al. Reparative effects of neural stem cells in neonatal rats with hypoxic-ischemic injury are not influenced by host sex. Pediatr Res. 2014;75(5):603–11. https://doi.org/10.1038/pr.2014.7.
32. Hsueh YY, Chang YJ, Huang CW, Handayani F, Chiang YL, Fan SC, et al. Synergy of endothelial and neural progenitor cells from adipose-derived stem cells to preserve neurovascular structures in rat hypoxic-ischemic brain injury. Sci Rep. 2015;5:14985. https://doi.org/10.1038/srep14985.
33. Luan Z, Liu W, Qu S, Du K, He S, Wang Z, et al. Effects of neural progenitor cell transplantation in children with severe cerebral palsy. Cell Transplant. 2012;21(Suppl 1):S91–8. https://doi.org/10.3727/096368912X633806.

Chapter 5
Hematopoietic Stem Cells for Perinatal Brain Injury

Masahiro Tsuji

Abstract Hematopoietic stem cells (HSCs) and cell fractions containing HSCs derived from bone marrow or umbilical cord blood have emerged as promising tools for cell-based therapies for perinatal brain injury. Nearly 20 studies in models of perinatal brain injury, most of which are rodent models of neonatal hypoxia-ischemia, have histologically and functionally demonstrated beneficial effects of systemic administration of HSCs and the related cell fraction. Studies have shown that the cell therapies are beneficial even if the cells are administered up to days after the insult. The cells do not directly differentiate into neurons or glial cells, nor do they regenerate damaged brain tissue. Instead, they elicit beneficial effects via other mechanisms, such as by modulating inflammatory/immune responses and increasing the levels of trophic factors, separate from their hematopoietic properties. Cell therapy with HSCs or the cell fraction containing HSCs has several advantages over other types of cell therapies. This approach does not require intracranial transplantation; intravenous transfusion seems sufficient for them to exert their beneficial effects. The cells are easily obtained, and neither gene manipulation nor cell culture is required. These advantages make HSC therapy feasible for translation into clinical use for infants with brain injury. The optimal protocol, however, has yet to be determined in further preclinical studies.

Keywords CD34-positive cell · Mononuclear cells · Umbilical cord blood cell
Neonatal brain damage

M. Tsuji, M.D., Ph.D.
Department of Regenerative Medicine and Tissue Engineering, National Cerebral and Cardiovascular Center, Suita, Osaka, Japan
e-mail: tsuji.masahiro.ri@ncvc.go.jp, mtsujimd@ybb.ne.jp

© Springer Nature Singapore Pte Ltd. 2018

H. Shintaku et al. (eds.), *Cell Therapy for Perinatal Brain Injury*,
https://doi.org/10.1007/978-981-10-1412-3_5

5.1 Introduction

Recently, hematopoietic stem cells (HSCs) have been considered a promising cell source for cell-based therapies for perinatal brain injury, in which neonatal hypoxic-ischemic encephalopathy (HIE) is the main pathophysiology. There are more than 20 reports of preclinical studies using HSCs to treat perinatal brain injuries (Table 5.1), and several clinical studies with HSCs are being conducted in patients with perinatal brain injuries (see Table 1.2 in Chap. 1). How did researchers and clinicians reach the idea that HSCs could be used for perinatal brain injuries? Two lines of thoughts likely lead to this approach. On the one hand, clinicians came to conceive that HSC transplantation (HSCT) might ameliorate brain injuries because of their successful experience with HSCT in patients with inborn errors of metabolism or neurodegenerative disorders. On the other hand, neuroscientists in the field of cell therapies came to think that HSCs might be a feasible alternative for cell-based therapy for brain injuries because other candidate cells have several problems to overcome before the clinical translation. Although transplanting neural stem cells (NSCs) into damaged cerebral tissue seems ideal for regenerating the brain after injury, obtaining the source cells for NSCs, such as embryonic stem (ES) cells, is difficult and ethically problematic. Additionally, obtaining uniform, high-quality NSCs is difficult, as differentiating into NSCs from ES cells requires elaborate techniques, and cultured NSCs often show tumorigenicity [1]. HSCs do not have the abovementioned issues. HSCs are abundant and readily available from bone marrow, peripheral blood, and umbilical cord blood; hence, there are no ethical problems with obtaining HSCs. Autologous cells are available as well, and in such cases, immunosuppression is not required for cell transplantation. Further, HSCs are not tumorigenic. Intravenous injection is the most feasible administration route for cell treatment. As HSCs exist physiologically in the blood stream, intravenous injection of HSCs is safe. Above all, HSCT has been used for the past few decades, and its safety has been demonstrated in infants and children.

5.2 History of Use of Hematopoietic Stem Cells in Clinical Practice

HSCs are the first and most common stem cells used in clinical practice. HSCT has been conducted for more than 5000 patients each year in Japan alone (Annual Report of Nationwide Survey 2013, The Japan Society for Hematopoietic Cell Transplantation). Although it was originally developed for and has been mainly conducted for patients with hematological diseases and malignancies, HSCT has also been performed for patients with inborn errors of metabolism or neurodegenerative disorders, for whom the basic purpose of the use of HSCs is enzyme/protein replacement. The reconstruction of the hematopoietic system with intact HSCs

Table 5.1 Review of reported studies in models with perinatal brain damage

	Research	Animal model		Cell			Timing [a]	Delivery	Follow-up	Improvement		Author and year
	Group	Age	Insult	Source	Type	Dose				Histology	Behavior	
1	A	P7 rat	HI	hUCB	MNC	1×10^7	24 h	i.p.	2 week	NA	Yes	Meier et al. [11]
2	A	P7 rat	HI	hUCB	MNC	1×10^7	24 h	i.p.	2 week	NA	NA	Rosenkranz et al. [31]
3	A	P7 rat	HI	hUCB	MNC	1×10^7	24 h	i.p.	6 week	Yes	NA	Geißler et al. [36]
4	A	P7 rat	HI	hUCB	MNC	1×10^7	24 h	i.p. or intrathecal	7 week	Yes	Yes	Wasielewski et al. [25]
5	A	P7 rat	HI	hUCB	MNC	1×10^7	24 h	i.p.	2 week	Yes	NA	Rosenkranz et al. [33]
6	A	P7 rat	HI	hUCB	MNC	1×10^7	24 h	i.p.	2 week	NA	NA	Rosenkranz et al. [35]
7	B	P7 rat	HI	hUCB	MNC	1×10^7	24 h	i.v.	3 week	No	No	De Paula et al. [12]
8	B	P7 rat	HI	hUCB	MNC	1×10^6, 10^7, 10^8	24 h	i.v.	8 week	Yes	Yes	De Paula [16]
9	B	P7 rat	HI	hUCB	MNC	1×10^6, 10^7	24 h	Intra-arterial	9 week	No	Yes	Greggio et al. [24]
10		P7 rat	HI	hUCB	MNC	1.5×10^4	7 day	i.v.	3 week	NA	Yes	Yasuhara et al. [37]
11		P7 rat	HI	hUCB	MNC	2×10^6	3 h	i.p.	7 day	Yes	Yes	Pimentel-Coelho et al. [34]
12		P7 rat	HI	hUCB	MNC	1×10^7	24 h	i.v.	10 week	Yes	Yes	Bae et al. [29]
13		P5 rat	Excitotoxicity	hUCB	MNC	1, 3×10^6, 1×10^7	0 h or 24 h	i.p. or i.v.	5 day	No	NA	Dalous et al. [13]
14	C	P7 rat	HI	hUCB	MNC	3×10^6	24 h	Intracranial	2 week	Yes	NA	Wang et al. [13]
15	C	P7 rat	HI	hUCB	MNC	3×10^6	24 h	Intracranial	4 week	Yes	NA	Wang et al. [14]
16	D	P12 mouse	pMCAO	hUCB	CD34+ cell	1×10^5	48 h	i.v.	7 week	Yes	No	Tsuji et al. [18]
17	D	P7 rat	HI	hUCB	MNC	1×10^7	6 h	i.p.	24 day	Yes	No	Hattori et al. [32]

(continued)

Table 5.1 (continued)

	Research	Animal model			Cell		Timing [a]	Delivery	Follow-up	Improvement		Author and year
	Group	Age	Insult	Source	Type	Dose				Histology	Behavior	
18		P14 rat	HI	hUCB	MNC	4×10^5	7 day	i.v.	14 day	Yes	Yes	Ghaffaripour et al. [22]
19		P12 mouse	pCCAO	hUCB	CD34+ enriched MNC	1×10^5	2 day	i.p.	4 week	No	No	Kadam et al. [17]
20		E22 rabbit	Uterine ischemia	hUCB	TNC	2.5 or 5×10^6	9 day	i.v.	20 day	NA	Yes	Drobyshevsky et al. [14]
21		P0 lamb	Uterine ischemia	Auto UCB	MNC	$\sim 1 \times 10^8$	12 h	Intra-arterial	72 h	Yes	NA	Aridas et al. [15]

Studies in which cells were administered before the brain injury are not included here

A–D, each alphabet indicates the same research group

P postnatal day, *E* embryonic day, *HI* hypoxia-ischemia, *pMCAO* permanent middle cerebral artery occlusion, *pCCAO* permanent common carotid artery occlusion, *hUCB* human umbilical cord blood, *auto* autologous, *MNC* mononuclear cell, CD34+ cell (hematopoietic stem/endothelial progenitor cell), *TNC* total nucleated cell, *i.p.* intraperitoneal *i.v.* intravenous, *NA* not assessed

Yes, at least one test among several tests examined is improved by the cell therapy, or at least one treatment protocol among several protocols tested is beneficial.

[a]Timing of the cell administration after injury

from a healthy donor supplies enzymes/proteins that are deficient in the recipient. HSCT has been shown to ameliorate neurodevelopmental deterioration in patients with adrenoleukodystrophy and mucopolysaccharidosis, such as Hurler and Hunter syndromes [2, 3]. Beneficial effects exerted by HSCT may not be exclusively derived from enzyme replacement. Autopsy studies demonstrated that donor cells can be identified in the brain and intestine months after the transplantation and that they contribute to new neurons and vascular endothelium [4, 5]. HSCT is considered to exert immunomodulatory effects in adrenoleukodystrophy via donor-derived microglia in the brain [6]. For patients with inborn errors of metabolism, allogeneic HSCs are used. Therefore, myeloablative treatment is required before the HSCT, and long-lasting immunosuppression is required after the HSCT. Those treatments associated with allogeneic cell transplantation often cause serious adverse effects, which can even be fatal. Autologous transplantation, in contrast, has no such adverse effects and is thus easier to conduct. After successful allogeneic HSCT for hundreds of children with inborn errors of metabolism, Kurtzberg and colleagues started autologous HSCT, intravenous administration of cryopreserved autologous umbilical cord blood (UCB), for patients with brain injuries other than inborn errors of metabolism, most of which were cerebral palsy [7]. They reported that autologous HSCT was feasible and safe.

5.3 History of Cell Therapies Using Hematopoietic Stem Cells in Animal Models with Perinatal Brain Injury

Dozens of preclinical studies on cell-based therapies for perinatal brain injuries have been reported after the first report of this kind in 1996, i.e., intracranial transplantation of neocortical tissue from fetal brain in a neonatal rat model [8]. During the first decade since that report, not more than ten studies were published. In all those studies, researchers transplanted NSCs or ES cells into the rodent brain in hopes that the transplanted cells would generate new neurons, replace lost neurons, and regenerate the damaged brain [9, 10]. The results were not favorable, as many of the transplanted cells do not survive or do survive but form tumors in the brain. Those studies indicated that several technical breakthroughs are required to translate those therapies, i.e., intracranial transplantation of neuronal lineage cells or multipotent stem cells, into clinical practice. Researchers sought a more feasible cell therapy for clinical use. Meier et al. presented the first report of beneficial effects of HSC therapy for perinatal brain injury in 2006 [11]. They administered the mononuclear cell (MNC) fraction of UCB intraperitoneally. Since then, more than 60 studies on cell therapies have been published in the field of perinatal brain injury research. Approximately one-third of those publications are studies using HSCs or the cell fraction containing HSCs.

5.4 Effects of Hematopoietic Stem Cells

Most of the published studies with HSCs or the cell fraction containing HSCs in models of perinatal brain injury have demonstrated benefits of the therapy. Some studies showed benefits in histological evaluations, others showed benefits in behavioral evaluation, and the others showed benefits in both evaluations. Although there may be publication bias in which negative results are less likely to be published, only two studies showed no benefit of HSC therapy [12, 13]. The beneficial effects of HSCs have been reported in several different disease models: neonatal HIE, neonatal stroke, excitotoxicity, and prenatal brain injury. All but two studies were conducted in rodent models; of those two, one was in rabbit [14] and the other in lamb [15].

5.5 Beneficial Cell Types for Perinatal Brain Injury

During the second decade of research in cell therapy for animal models with perinatal brain injury, i.e., from 2006 onward, bone marrow (BM) and UCB have been the major cell sources, and MNCs and mesenchymal stem cells (MSCs) have been the major cell types to be administered. MSCs are derived from various tissues including BM and UCB, and they do not contain HSCs, while BM- or UCB-derived MNCs contain HSCs as their major stem cell type. MNCs are easily isolated from BM and UCB by gradient centrifugation. HSCs form 0.1 to 2% of a BM- or UCB-derived MNC fraction, and lymphocytes form the majority of the fraction [7, 16]. UCB is used as a cell source to collect HSCs or MNCs in almost all preclinical studies. BM-derived HSCs or MNCs are used frequently in studies on adult brain injury but not in studies on perinatal brain injury. Preferential use of UCB in perinatal studies may be due to the high availability of autologous UCB when translated into clinical practice, whereas autologous UCB is not available in many adult cases. A more purified HSC fraction, which is $CD34^+$ cells of human UCB ($CD34^+$ is a cell-surface marker for HSCs/endothelial progenitor cells), has been examined only in two studies [17, 18]. Studies have shown that either cell type, MNCs or $CD34^+$ cells, is beneficial for perinatal brain injury. No study has ever directly compared the effects of the $CD34^+$ cells with MNCs in perinatal brain injury models. Therefore, it is not known whether HSCs are the only cell type beneficial for brain injury. A few studies in a model of adult stroke compared the effects of different cell types. In one study, human UCB-$CD34^+$ cells, but not $CD34^-$ cells, ameliorated the brain damage [19]. In another study, human UCB-MNCs (which include $CD34^+$ cells) provided the most marked neuroprotective effects, followed by $CD34^+$ cells only, and $CD34^-$ cells were least effective [20]. In a clinical study of adult patients with stroke, a higher number of circulating $CD34^+$ cells in peripheral blood was associated with better functional recovery [21]. Those results suggest that $CD34^+$ cells have a crucial role in neuroprotection and neurological recovery.

All studies in rodents with UCB cells were xenotransplantation, i.e., human cells were transfused to rodents. A recent study used autologous UCB-MNCs in a lamb model, and the treatment was shown to be neuroprotective [15].

5.6 Therapeutic Time Window of HSCs

People tend to consider regenerative properties as the most attractive characteristics of cell therapies. I, however, consider the long therapeutic time window to be just as attractive as the regenerative properties. Almost all therapies proven effective in preclinical studies have very short time windows in which to exert their effects either in neonatal models or in adult models. Many treatments exert their beneficial effects only when administered before brain injury. Although some treatments show neuroprotective effects even when administered after the insult, the time window rarely exceeds 4 h after the insult. Only a very few treatments showed benefits when administered more than 24 h after brain injury. In stark contrast, most cell therapies demonstrated beneficial effects even if the cells were administered more than 24 h after brain injury. UCB cell therapies have been shown to be effective when cells were administered 7 days after the insult in a neonatal HIE model [22] and as late as 30 days after the insult in an adult stroke model [23]. Notably, in contrast to the growing evidence of cell therapies for the acute and subacute phases of perinatal brain injuries, no study has focused on the chronic phase of perinatal brain injuries. Therefore, there is no preclinical evidence regarding cell therapies for children or teenagers with brain injuries that originated in the perinatal period.

5.7 Optimal Cell Dose of HSCs

Preclinical studies demonstrated beneficial effects of administration of HSCs or HSC-containing cells, but the cell doses varied widely depending on the study: from 1.5×10^4 up to 1×10^8 cells/rodent. The optimal dose may depend on various factors, such as the cell type, the type and severity of insult, the route of administration, and the timing of the treatment. Four studies examined different cell doses. de Paula et al. compared three different doses, 1×10^6, 1×10^7, and 1×10^8 human UCB-MNCs, administered intravenously in a rat model of neonatal HIE and found that only the highest dose produced significant improvement in spatial learning impairment and that the highest and medium doses produced significant improvement in cerebral volume loss [16]. The same research group compared two different doses, 1×10^6 and 1×10^7 human UCB-MNCs, administered intra-arterially in the same model and found that only the higher dose produced significant improvement in spatial learning impairment [24]. Dalous et al. compared three different doses, 1×10^6, 3×10^6, and 1×10^7 human UCB-MNCs administered intravenously or intraperitoneally in a neonatal rat model of excitotoxic brain injury and evaluated at 5 days after the insult [13]. Neither cell dose was beneficial when administered intravenously, while the highest dose was detrimental by activating systemic inflammation when administered intraperitoneally. Drobyshevsky et al. examined two different doses, 2.5×10^6 and 5×10^6 human UCB-MNCs, administered intravenously in a rabbit model of intrauterine ischemia [14]. Either dose ameliorated motor impairment, although the lower dose showed lesser improvement. Taken together, as far as intravenous injection is concerned, high doses, such as 1×10^7 cells, seem safe and more beneficial for brain injury. Further studies are needed to find the optimal cell doses for each specific medical condition.

5.8 Route of Administration

Most researchers administered HSCs and HSC-containing cell fractions systemically, i.e., intravenously or intraperitoneally, rather than intracranially. Only few studies examined the effects of local transplantation [25–27]. Two studies from the same research group showed that intracranial transplantation of human UCB-MNCs ameliorates brain injury. As those cells are blood cells, intravenous administration is theoretically physiological and noninvasive and is hence a feasible route for clinical use. The intraperitoneal route is commonly used as an alternative to the intravenous route for administering chemical compounds in neonatal rodents, as intraperitoneal injection is easier than intravenous injection. In nearly half of published studies on neonatal brain injury, cells were administered intraperitoneally. When administering cells, however, the intraperitoneal route is not comparable to intravenous one. We reported that cell distributions in the body are different depending on the routes of administration, as well as depending on the cell types [28]. A small percentage of MNCs infused either intravenously or intraperitoneally were identified in the rodent brains; instead, intravenously administered cells were localized in the lungs, liver, and spleen. The same was true in nonhuman primates. In contrast, intraperitoneally administered cells were found in those organs in low numbers. Only one study, apart from that of Dalous et al., compared the effects of different routes of administration. Wasielewski et al. showed human UCB-MNCs administered either intraperitoneally or intrathecally were equally beneficial [25]. Intra-arterial transfusion into the carotid artery seems to be an attractive route of cell administration as the cells are delivered directly to the brain via the blood stream. A research group reported separately the effects of mostly similar cell therapies but with different routes of administration: one was intravenous injection, and the other was intra-arterial injection via the contralateral common carotid artery [16, 24]. The cell therapies seemed equally beneficial via either route of administration; in other words, intra-arterial delivery did not appear superior to intravenous delivery. Overall, data are scarce regarding which route of administration is the most effective. Nevertheless, considering the safety and feasibility for use in sick infants, the intravenous route may be the optimal one. A body of evidence has shown that long-term survival of a high number of administered cells in the brain is not always necessary to exert beneficial effects. Quite a few studies demonstrated beneficial effects despite few [14, 18, 29] or even no transfused cells were found in the brain [20, 30]. Other studies showed that infused cells migrate to the lesion site, in a phenomenon called "homing," attracted by some sort of signal, such as the chemokine stromal-derived factor (SDF)-1 (CXCL12) [31]. Due to the possibility of homing, direct cell delivery to the brain may not be necessary. Taken together, intravenous administration may be the optimal route from the standpoints of both efficacy and safety.

5.9 Mechanisms of Action

Mechanisms of cell therapies with HSCs and HSC-containing blood cell fractions are multifaceted. Studies have shown several different mechanisms of action in ameliorating and improving neonatal brain injury. My collaborators and our laboratory found that UCB-HSCs ($CD34^+$ cells) ameliorate reduced blood flow around the ischemic lesion [18] and that UCB-MNCs reduce oxidative stress and apoptosis in the lesioned brain [32]. Reduction of apoptosis by UCB-MNCs has also been reported by Rosenkranz et al. [33]. Transfusion of human UCB-MNCs reduces HI-induced inflammatory responses in the brain, i.e., microglia infiltration and astrocytic activation [25, 32, 34], although a study reported that cell transfusion causes a transient increase in microglia [29]. In addition, cell transfusion reduces systemic inflammatory responses, such as reducing the elevated serum level of interleukin-1α [35]. Bae et al. demonstrated that human UCB-MNCs increase the levels of CCL3/macrophage inflammatory protein 1α (MIP-1α) in the injured brain (2012). Their in vitro study, however, showed that the cells secrete low levels of CCL3/MIP-1α but high levels of several other cytokines, which do not show increases in the brain after the cell transfusion. Interaction between donor cells and the recipient may determine the levels of cytokines and trophic factors in the brain and peripheral blood [29]. Transplantation of human UCB-MNCs promotes endogenous NSC proliferation via the sonic hedgehog signaling pathway [26]. Electrophysiological studies have demonstrated that human UCB-MNCs ameliorate HI-induced hyperexcitability as well as distorted cortical maps and receptive fields [36]. UCB-MNCs increase the levels of several trophic factors, i.e., GDNF, NGF, BDNF, and VEGF, as well as expression of the proteins tie-2 and occludin, in the brain [33, 37]. As VEGF and the angiopoietin-1/tie-2 system are crucial for angiogenesis, UCB-MNC transfusion may cause growth of blood vessels in the injured brain. As occludin is an integral component of the blood-brain barrier, the cell administration may contribute to reconstruction of the blood-brain barrier. In summary, HSCs and HSC-containing blood cell fractions exert multiple beneficial effects that are not directly related to hematopoietic capacity. This multifaceted nature of these stem cells may be one of the advantages of cell-based therapies.

5.10 Conclusions

Accumulating evidence from preclinical studies shows that systemic administration of HSCs and HSC-containing blood cell fractions have potential to ameliorate perinatal brain injury, even when transfused hours or days after the insult. Systemic administration of human UCB-MNCs is the most extensively explored therapy, and many studies from several laboratories have demonstrated its beneficial effects. From a clinical perspective, intravenous transfusion of autologous UCB-MNCs is the most feasible and has the lowest risk for adverse events when used in infants with brain injury. Few studies, however, have examined different treatment protocols; hence, the optimal protocol is not yet known. Further preclinical studies are warranted.

References

1. Comi AM, Cho E, Mulholland JD, Hooper A, Li Q, Qu Y, et al. Neural stem cells reduce brain injury after unilateral carotid ligation. Pediatr Neurol. 2008;38:86–92.
2. Peters C, Shapiro EG, Anderson J, Henslee-Downey PJ, Klemperer MR, Cowan MJ, et al. Hurler syndrome: II. Outcome of HLA-genotypically identical sibling and HLA-haploidentical related donor bone marrow transplantation in fifty-four children. The storage disease collaborative study group. Blood. 1998;91:2601–8.
3. Aldenhoven M, Kurtzberg J. Cord blood is the optimal graft source for the treatment of pediatric patients with lysosomal storage diseases: clinical outcomes and future directions. Cytotherapy. 2015;17:765–74.
4. Mezey E, Key S, Vogelsang G, Szalayova I, Lange GD, Crain B. Transplanted bone marrow generates new neurons in human brains. Proc Natl Acad Sci U S A. 2003;100:1364–9.
5. Jiang S, Walker L, Afentoulis M, Anderson DA, Jauron-Mills L, Corless CL, et al. Transplanted human bone marrow contributes to vascular endothelium. Proc Natl Acad Sci U S A. 2004;101:16891–6.
6. Moser HW, Mahmood A. New insights about hematopoietic stem cell transplantation in adrenoleukodystrophy. Arch Neurol. 2007;64:631–2.
7. Sun J, Allison J, McLaughlin C, Sledge L, Waters-Pick B, Wease S, et al. Differences in quality between privately and publicly banked umbilical cord blood units: a pilot study of autologous cord blood infusion in children with acquired neurologic disorders. Transfusion. 2010;50:1980–7.
8. Elsayed MH, Hogan TP, Shaw PL, Castro AJ. Use of fetal cortical grafts in hypoxic-ischemic brain injury in neonatal rats. Exp Neurol. 1996;137:127–41.
9. Park KI, Teng YD, Snyder EY. The injured brain interacts reciprocally with neural stem cells supported by scaffolds to reconstitute lost tissue. Nat Biotechnol. 2002;20:1111–7.
10. Vadivelu S, Platik MM, Choi L, Lacy ML, Shah AR, Qu Y, et al. Multi-germ layer lineage central nervous system repair: nerve and vascular cell generation by embryonic stem cells transplanted in the injured brain. J Neurosurg. 2005;103:124–35.
11. Meier C, Middelanis J, Wasielewski B, Neuhoff S, Roth-Haerer A, Gantert M, et al. Spastic paresis after perinatal brain damage in rats is reduced by human cord blood mononuclear cells. Pediatr Res. 2006;59:244–9.
12. de Paula S, Vitola AS, Greggio S, de Paula D, Mello PB, Lubianca JM, et al. Hemispheric brain injury and behavioral deficits induced by severe neonatal hypoxia-ischemia in rats are not attenuated by intravenous administration of human umbilical cord blood cells. Pediatr Res. 2009;65:631–5.

13. Dalous J, Pansiot J, Pham H, Chatel P, Nadaradja C, D'Agostino I, et al. Use of human umbilical cord blood mononuclear cells to prevent perinatal brain injury: a preclinical study. Stem Cells Dev. 2012;22:169–79.
14. Drobyshevsky A, Cotten CM, Shi Z, Luo K, Jiang R, Derrick M, et al. Human umbilical cord blood cells ameliorate motor deficits in rabbits in a cerebral palsy model. Dev Neurosci. 2015;37:349–62.
15. Aridas JD, McDonald CA, Paton MC, Yawno T, Sutherland AE, et al. Cord blood mononuclear cells prevent neuronal apoptosis in response to perinatal asphyxia in the newborn lamb. J Physiol. 2016;594:1421–35.
16. de Paula S, Greggio S, Marinowic DR, Machado DC, DaCosta JC. The dose-response effect of acute intravenous transplantation of human umbilical cord blood cells on brain damage and spatial memory deficits in neonatal hypoxia-ischemia. Neuroscience. 2012;210:431–41.
17. Kadam SD, Chen H, Markowitz GJ, Raja S, George S, Verina T, et al. Systemic injection of CD34(+)-enriched human cord blood cells modulates poststroke neural and glial response in a sex-dependent manner in CD1 mice. Stem Cells Dev. 2015;24:51–66.
18. Tsuji M, Taguchi A, Ohshima M, Kasahara Y, Sato Y, Tsuda H, et al. Effects of intravenous administration of umbilical cord blood CD34(+) cells in a mouse model of neonatal stroke. Neuroscience. 2014;263:148–58.
19. Taguchi A, Soma T, Tanaka H, Kanda T, Nishimura H, Yoshikawa H, et al. Administration of CD34+ cells after stroke enhances neurogenesis via angiogenesis in a mouse model. J Clin Invest. 2004;114:330–8.
20. Boltze J, Reich DM, Hau S, Reymann KG, Strassburger M, Lobsien D, et al. Assessment of neuroprotective effects of human umbilical cord blood mononuclear cell subpopulations in vitro and in vivo. Cell Transplant. 2012;21:723–37.
21. Dunac A, Frelin C, Popolo-Blondeau M, Chatel M, Mahagne MH, Philip PJ. Neurological and functional recovery in human stroke are associated with peripheral blood CD34+ cell mobilization. J Neurol. 2007;254:327–32.
22. Ghaffaripour HA, Jalali M, Nikravesh MR, Seghatoleslam M, Sanchooli J. Neuronal cell reconstruction with umbilical cord blood cells in the brain hypoxia-ischemia. Iran Biomed J. 2015;19:29–34.
23. Zhang L, Li Y, Zhang C, Chopp M, Gosiewska A, Hong K. Delayed administration of human umbilical tissue-derived cells improved neurological functional recovery in a rodent model of focal ischemia. Stroke. 2011;42:1437–44.
24. Greggio S, de Paula S, Azevedo PN, Venturin GT, Dacosta JC. Intra-arterial transplantation of human umbilical cord blood mononuclear cells in neonatal hypoxic-ischemic rats. Life Sci. 2014;96:33–9.
25. Wasielewski B, Jensen A, Roth-Harer A, Dermietzel R, Meier C. Neuroglial activation and Cx43 expression are reduced upon transplantation of human umbilical cord blood cells after perinatal hypoxic-ischemic injury. Brain Res. 2012;1487:39–53.
26. Wang XL, Zhao YS, Hu MY, Sun YQ, Chen YX, Bi XH. Umbilical cord blood cells regulate endogenous neural stem cell proliferation via hedgehog signaling in hypoxic ischemic neonatal rats. Brain Res. 2013;1518:26–35.
27. Wang X, Zhao Y, Wang X. Umbilical cord blood cells regulate the differentiation of endogenous neural stem cells in hypoxic ischemic neonatal rats via the hedgehog signaling pathway. Brain Res. 2014;1560:18–26.
28. Ohshima M, Taguchi A, Tsuda H, Sato Y, Yamahara K, Harada-Shiba M, et al. Intraperitoneal and intravenous deliveries are not comparable in terms of drug efficacy and cell distribution in neonatal mice with hypoxia-ischemia. Brain and Development. 2015;37:376–86.
29. Bae SH, Lee HS, Kang MS, Strupp BJ, Chopp M, Moon J. The levels of pro-inflammatory factors are significantly decreased in cerebral palsy patients following an allogeneic umbilical cord blood cell transplant. Int J Stem Cells. 2012;5:31–8.
30. Borlongan CV, Hadman M, Sanberg CD, Sanberg PR. Central nervous system entry of peripherally injected umbilical cord blood cells is not required for neuroprotection in stroke. Stroke. 2004;35:2385–9.

31. Rosenkranz K, Kumbruch S, Lebermann K, Marschner K, Jensen A, Dermietzel R, et al. The chemokine SDF-1/CXCL12 contributes to the 'homing' of umbilical cord blood cells to a hypoxic-ischemic lesion in the rat brain. J Neurosci Res. 2010;88:1223–33.
32. Hattori T, Sato Y, Kondo T, Ichinohashi Y, Sugiyama Y, Yamamoto M, et al. Administration of umbilical cord blood cells transiently decreased hypoxic-ischemic brain injury in neonatal rats. Dev Neurosci. 2015;37:95–104.
33. Rosenkranz K, Kumbruch S, Tenbusch M, Marcus K, Marschner K, Dermietzel R, et al. Transplantation of human umbilical cord blood cells mediated beneficial effects on apoptosis, angiogenesis and neuronal survival after hypoxic-ischemic brain injury in rats. Cell Tissue Res. 2012;348:429–38.
34. Pimentel-Coelho PM, Magalhaes ES, Lopes LM, deAzevedo LC, Santiago MF, Mendez-Otero R. Human cord blood transplantation in a neonatal rat model of hypoxic-ischemic brain damage: functional outcome related to neuroprotection in the striatum. Stem Cells Dev. 2010;19:351–8.
35. Rosenkranz K, Tenbusch M, May C, Marcus K, Meier C. Changes in Interleukin-1 alpha serum levels after transplantation of umbilical cord blood cells in a model of perinatal hypoxic-ischemic brain damage. Ann Anat. 2013;195:122–7.
36. Geißler M, Dinse HR, Neuhoff S, Kreikemeier K, Meier C. Human umbilical cord blood cells restore brain damage induced changes in rat somatosensory cortex. PLoS One. 2011;6:e20194.
37. Yasuhara T, Hara K, Maki M, Xu L, Yu G, Ali MM, et al. Mannitol facilitates neurotrophic factor up-regulation and behavioural recovery in neonatal hypoxic-ischaemic rats with human umbilical cord blood grafts. J Cell Mol Med. 2010;14:914–21.

Chapter 6
Umbilical Cord-Derived Mesenchymal Stromal Cells for Perinatal Brain Injury

Tokiko Nagamura-Inoue and Takeo Mukai

Abstract Recently, umbilical cord (UC)-derived mesenchymal stromal cells (UC-MSCs) have become an attractive cell source in regenerative medicine for many reasons including (1) no adverse events during collection, (2) ease of collection even after cord blood (CB) collection or failure to collect CB, (3) minimal ethical controversy, (4) multipotency to differentiate into various cell types, and (5) low immunogenicity with significant immunosuppressive ability. In this chapter, we provide a brief introduction of UC and UC-MSC characteristics, isolation, and cryopreservation and emphasize their potential clinical application for neurological disorders, especially perinatal brain injury.

Keywords Mesenchymal stromal cells · Umbilical cord · Perinatal brain injury Neurogenic differentiation

6.1 Introduction

The use of human mesenchymal stromal cells (MSCs) to treat various diseases has recently been investigated. MSCs can be harvested from various tissues, including the bone marrow (BM) [1], cord blood (CB) [2], adipose tissue [3], placenta [4], and umbilical cord (UC) [5].

T. Nagamura-Inoue, M.D., Ph.D. (✉)
Department of Cell Processing and Transfusion, Research Hospital, The Institute of Medical Science, The University of Tokyo, Tokyo, Japan
e-mail: tokikoni@ims.u-tokyo.ac.jp

T. Mukai, M.D., Ph.D.
Division of Molecular Therapy, Center for Advanced Medical Research, The Institute of Medical Science, The University of Tokyo, Tokyo, Japan

© Springer Nature Singapore Pte Ltd. 2018
H. Shintaku et al. (eds.), *Cell Therapy for Perinatal Brain Injury*,
https://doi.org/10.1007/978-981-10-1412-3_6

The UC links the mother and fetus during pregnancy, but it is fated to become medical waste soon after delivery. The UC normally contains two umbilical arteries and one umbilical vein buried in Wharton's jelly (WJ), from which fibroblast-like cells (MSCs) are isolated. Since the first description of UC-MSCs in 1991 by McElreavey et al. [6], many reports have demonstrated that UC-derived MSCs (UC-MSCs) have multipotency and self-renewal properties comparable to MSCs derived from other tissues. Here, we focus on UC-MSCs as a great alternative MSC source with several advantages, especially for prenatal babies. These advantages include (1) no adverse events during the collection process, (2) ease of collection even after CB collection or failure to collect CB, (3) minimal ethical controversy, (4) multipotent ability to differentiate into various cell types, and (5) low immunogenicity with significant immunosuppressive ability.

UC-MSCs have attracted considerable interest because of their immunomodulatory properties. They express less human leukocyte antigen (HLA) class II even in the presence of inflammation cytokines such as interferon (IFN-γ) [7] and are thus less immunogenic. In recent years, UC-MSCs have been proposed as a multipurpose tool for regenerative medicine and immunotherapy.

Here, we describe UC-MSCs including present isolation and cryopreservation methods. We also propose their potential clinical application for neurological disorders, especially perinatal brain injury.

6.2 UC-MSC Isolation Methods

There are diverse protocols and culture methods for isolating MSCs from the various UC compartments such as WJ, vein, arteries, UC lining membrane, subamnion, and perivascular regions. The specific isolation methods have been described elsewhere [8].

We review two major isolation approaches: the explants and enzymatic digestion methods. In the former, UC is collected and manually minced into small 1–2 mm^3 fragments. These fragments are aligned and regularly seeded on a tissue culture-treated dish. Once the tissue fragments attach to the bottom of the dish, culture media is slowly and gently added to avoid detachment [9–11]. When fibroblast-like adherent cells reach 80–90% confluence in 2–4 weeks, adherent cells and tissue fragments are detached using trypsin. The culture is then filtered to remove tissue fragments. Unfortunately, tissue fragments often float in the media, resulting in the poor cell recovery. To prevent exfoliation of tissue fragments from the bottom of the culture dish, we employed a stainless steel mesh (Cellamigo®; Tsubakimoto Chain Co.) to prevent tissue fragments from floating. In this manner, we could plate source tissue more quickly and harvest more MSCs. In addition, this method also reduced the incubation time required to reach 80–90% confluence [12].

In the latter enzymatic explants method, the UC is minced into small pieces and immersed in media containing enzymes such as collagenase or a combination of collagenase and hyaluronidase with or without trypsin [9, 13, 14]. Tissues are then incubated with shaking for 2–3 h, washed with media, and seeded on a tissue culture-treated dish. MSCs are then obtained as previously described [9–11].

6.3 UC and UC-MSC Cryopreservation

There are several reports of UC tissue cryopreservation using serum-free and xenogeneic animal-free (xeno-free) cryoprotectants. Ennis et al. introduced CryoStor® (Stemcell Technologies Inc., Canada) for isolating human UC perivascular cells (HUPVCs), although they did not show the comparative test results [15]. Roy et al. described UC tissue cryopreservation in 10% dimethyl sulfoxide and 0.2 M sucrose solution, but the cumulative cell yield derived from the frozen-thawed UC-MSCs in their solution was inferior to that of fresh UC-MSCs [16]. We recently reported a UC tissue cryopreservation method with no impact on viability using a serum- and animal origin-free cryoprotectant, STEM-CELLBANKER® [17].

Our institution currently cryopreserves and thaws UC and UC-MSCs for use in research because of the possibility that cryopreservation and thawing UC and UC-MSCs will be required for both allogeneic and autologous administration in future clinical applications.

6.4 UC-MSC Characteristics

The Mesenchymal and Tissue Stem Cell Committee of the International Society for Cellular Therapy (ISCT) proposed minimal criteria for defining human MSCs [18, 19]. First, MSCs must be plastic adherent when maintained in standard culture conditions. Second, MSC must express CD105, CD73, and CD90 but not CD45, CD34, CD14/CD11b, CD79α/CD19, or HLA-DR surface molecules. Third, MSCs can differentiate into adipocytes, chondroblasts, and osteoblasts in vitro, although UC-MSC osteogenic differentiation is not well understood.

6.4.1 Biomarkers

UC-MSCs isolated from specific areas of the UC and whole cord satisfy the biomarker criteria defined by the Mesenchymal and Tissue Stem Cell Committee of the ISCT [18, 19]. Thus, UC-MSCs are positive for CD73, CD90, and CD105; low positive for HLA class I; and negative for the hematopoietic, macrophage, and endothelial markers CD14, 19, 31, 34, and 45 and HLA class II [20]. In addition, the Oct4 and Sox2 transcription factors essential for pluripotency and self-renewal are initially expressed at low levels but gradually decrease with repeated passage [21]. In addition, Guo et al. revealed that spheroid culture increases multipotency and alters the epigenetic status of pluripotency genes, resulting in higher Oct4, Sox2, and Nanog expression [22].

6.4.2 Immunosuppressive Properties

Immunosuppressive effects are the most promising property of MSCs for their potential clinical use [8]. Defective HLA class II expression in UC-MSCs can theoretically rescue them from immune recognition by CD4+ T cells [23]. Moreover, MSCs do not express co-stimulatory surface antigens that activate T cells, such as CD40, CD80, or CD86 [24]. Thus, MSCs escape activated T cells and exert immunomodulatory effects.

MSCs can inhibit immune cell proliferation and cytokine secretion, as well as alter subtypes in vitro [25–28]. The immunomodulation may be linked to soluble factors such as indoleamine 2,3-dioxygenase (IDO), prostaglandin E2, galectin-1, HLA-G5 [29], hepatocyte growth factor, interleukin-10, and transforming growth factor-β1 released from MSCs [30]. On the other hand, several studies have reported that UC-MSCs may only display immunosuppressive properties following exposure to inflammatory cytokines and/or activated T cells, a process called licensing or priming [31–33]. In this context, Deuse et al. reported that a high IFN-γ enhanced immunosuppression by further elevating IDO production [32]. HLA class II induction by IFN-γ is well-known in BM-MSCs, but it is controversial in UC-MSCs. Recently, Han et al. reported that IL-17 dramatically enhanced the immunosuppressive effect of MSCs induced by IFN-γ and tumor necrosis factor (TNF)-α [34]. These results indicate that priming may be a suitable therapeutic application. Nevertheless, the specific mechanisms of immune modulation by UC-MSCs remain undefined.

6.4.3 In Vitro Differentiation into Osteoblasts, Adipocytes, and Chondrocytes

UC-MSCs are multipotent and differentiate into various cell types including osteoblasts, adipocytes, and chondroblasts [35–37]. However, lipid accumulation is much slower in UC-MSCs during adipogenesis and produces adipocytes less mature than those derived from BM [36]. Mennan et al. reported that UC-MSCs produce small lipid vacuoles, whereas BM-MSCs produce more mature adipocytes with unilocular lipid vacuoles [20]. A possible reason is that UC-MSCs retain multipotency longer than MSCs derived from BM [38].

Conversely, UC-MSCs have been reported to have abundant potential to differentiate into chondroblasts [12, 20]. UC-MSCs produce three times as much collagen as BM-MSCs, suggesting that they may be better sources for engineering fibrocartilage [39].

The ability of UC-MSCs to differentiate into osteoblasts remains controversial. Hsieh et al. demonstrated that UC-MSCs show delayed and incomplete differentiation. This could be because BM-MSCs are more similar to osteoblasts and thus have better osteogenic potential [40], while UC-MSCs are more primitive and share more common genes with embryonic stem cells [41].

6.5 Potential to Differentiate into Neural Cells *In Vitro*

In addition to adipocytes, chondrocytes, and osteoblasts, several studies have demonstrated the potential of MSCs to differentiate into cells resembling neural stem cells [42, 43]. Hsieh et al. reported that WJ-derived MSCs expressed more genes, especially secreted factors, involved in angiogenesis and neurogenesis; functional validation showed that WJ-MSCs induced better neural differentiation and neural cell migration via a paracrine mechanism [44]. We also reported the neurogenic differentiation potentials of UC-MSCs and UC-MSCs after neurosphere formation (UC-MSC-neurospheres) [45]. Both were capable of differentiating into neurogenic cells when cultured in neurogenic differentiation medium (Fig. 6.1). However, preconditioned UC-MSC-neurospheres exhibited significantly higher neural marker expression compared with those directly derived from UC-MSCs. Therefore,

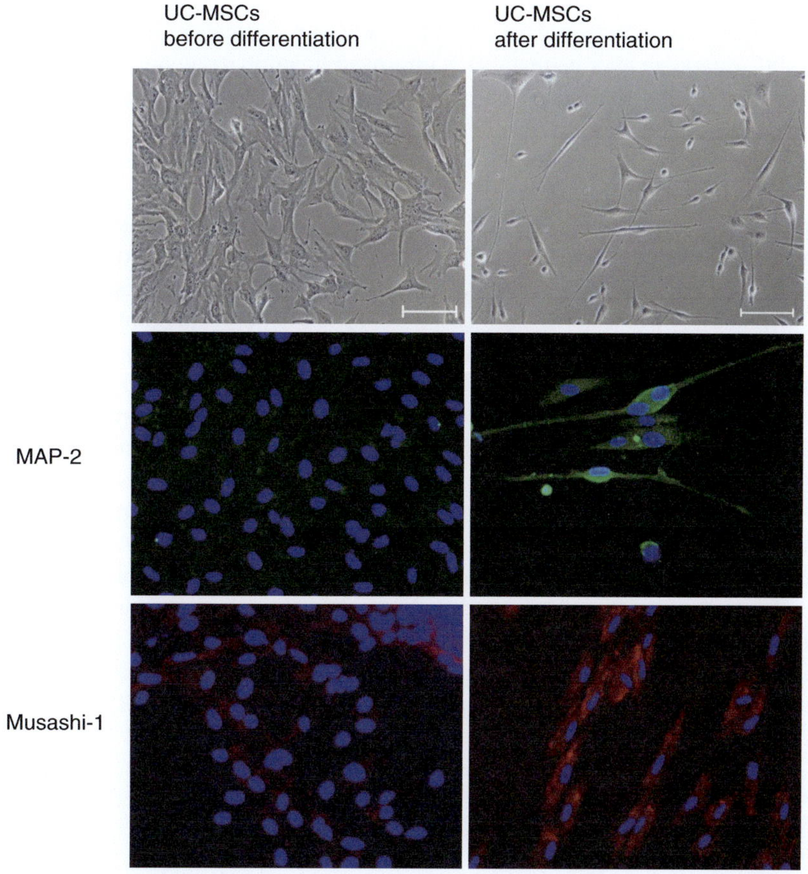

Fig. 6.1 Neurogenic differentiation of UC-MSCs. UC-MSCs shifted to a neuronal-like bipolar morphology with long thin processes in response to culturing in neurogenic differentiation medium (**a**, **b**), and there were more MAP-2 (**c**, **d**)- and MUSASHI-1 (**e**, **f**)-positive cells in differentiated UC-MSCs compared to their undifferentiated counterparts (scale bar = 100 μm)

neurogenic differentiation potential is probably greater in UC-MSC-neurospheres, although both UC-MSCs and UC-MSC-neurospheres may serve as useful cell sources for neurogenic regenerative medicine.

6.6 UC-MSCs in a Perinatal Brain Injury Animal Model

Hypoxic-ischemic encephalopathy (HIE), also known as neonatal encephalopathy, is a common perinatal medical problem throughout the world. The reported incidence of HIE in developed countries is approximately 1–4 per 1000 live term births. It is a major cause of postnatal death and permanent neurodevelopmental disabilities, especially cerebral palsy [46]. During hypoxic-ischemic brain injury, neurons and glial cells are damaged and lose functionality or die. Recent advances in regenerative medicine suggest that stem cell transplantation, especially MSCs, may help repair the damaged brain. With regard to BM-MSCs, van Velthoven et al. reported that BM-MSC treatment after neonatal HIE improved functional outcome, reduced lesion volume, increased differentiation of recently divided cells toward neurons and oligodendrocytes, and decreased proliferating inflammatory cells [47]. Jellema et al. described neuroprotective and anti-inflammatory effects of intravenously delivered BM-MSCs in an ovine model of HIE. They reported that BM-MSCs reduced microglial proliferation, attenuated oligodendrocyte loss, reduced demyelination in the preterm brain, induced persistent peripheral T-cell tolerance in vivo, and reduced invasion of T cells into the preterm brain following global hypoxic ischemia [48].

Other studies have tested the effects of UC-MSCs in perinatal brain injury models. Ding et al. reported that UC-MSC transplantation significantly alleviated ischemic injury in a mouse model of middle cerebral artery occlusion (MCAO). The rescue is the result of differentiation of transplanted cells into neurons and astrocytes, thereby enhancing plasticity [49]. Zhu et al. reported that UC-MSC transplantation improves glial cell function in cerebral white matter and enhances long-term behavioral function in a rat model of periventricular white matter damage [50]. Cheng et al. suggested that UC-MSCs have neuroprotective effects in mice after MCAO, presumably by transforming growth factor-β modulation of peripheral immune-inflammation [51]. Our recent investigation agreed with those reports, showing that intravenously administered UC-MSCs migrate towards the brain and attenuate intraventricular hemorrhage induced injuries secreting neurotrophic factors such as brain-derived neurotrophic factor (BDNF) and hepatocyte growth factor (HGF) [52].

Collectively, the results of these experiments strongly suggest that UC-MSC transplantation has powerful therapeutic potential for perinatal brain injury.

6.7 Clinical Applications for Neurological Disorders

Use of off-the-shelf UC-MSCs from an allogeneic third party is limited except in special circumstances such as perinatal injuries. Data from clinical trials using allogeneic third-party UC-MSCs or WJ-MSCs for neurological disorders with favorable results have recently been published and are summarized in Table 6.1.

Table 6.1 Summary of clinical trials using umbilical cord-derived mesenchymal stromal cells for neurological disorders

Disease	Number of patients	Mean age (range), year	Administration route	Number of cells	Number of injections	Results	Adverse events	Reference
SCA/MSA-C	14/10	46	IT	1×10^6/kg at 7-day interval	4	Delayed progression of neurological deficits	Dizziness, back pain, headache	Dongmei et al. [57]
Hereditary SCA	16	39.9 (21–56)	IV + IT	IV: 4×10^7 IT: 2×10^7 cells at 7-day interval	4	Motor functional recovery after 6 months	No	Jin et al. [58]
Traumatic brain injury	20	27.5 (5–48)	IT	1×10^7 at 5–7-day interval	4	Motor functional recovery after 6 months	No	Wang et al. [59]
Cerebral palsy	16 (8 twins)	6.29 (3–12)	IT	1–1.5×10^7 cells at 3–5-day interval	4	Motor functional recovery after 1 and 6 months	No	Wang et al. [60]

Modified table from [61]
IT intrathecal injection, *IV* intravenous injection, *SCA/MSA-C* spinocerebellar ataxia and multiple system atrophy-cerebellar type

There are many reports of using BM-MSCs to treat central nervous system disorders [53–56]. For example, Wang et al. demonstrated that BM-MSC transplantation is safe and has a clear reconditioning effect in the setting of spinal cord injury, probably via nerve cell trophism, immunosuppression, and axonal regeneration [56].

Clinical trials of UC-MSCs to treat central nervous system injuries have begun and are rapidly increasing in number. Dongmei et al. described intrathecal UC-MSC injection to delay progression of spinocerebellar ataxia and multiple system atrophy-cerebellar type [57]. The injections improved patient symptoms and scores on the International Cooperative Ataxia Rating Scale (ICARS). Dizziness, headache, and back pain that resolved within 1–3 days were the only reported side effects. Jin et al. [58] also described trials in which UC-MSCs were used to treat hereditary spinocerebellar ataxia. There were no serious adverse transplant-related events, and the majority of patients showed improved scores on the Berg Balance Scale and ICARS. On the other hand, Wang [59] demonstrated the potential of UC-MSCs to treat traumatic brain injuries. Most recently, Wang et al. [60] described the impact of UC-MSC transplantation on the motor function of identical twins with cerebral palsy. Eight pairs of twins showed significantly improved Gross Motor Function Measures at 1 and 6 months after therapy.

The clinical improvements observed following UC-MSCs administration for neurological disorders suggest that UC-MSC therapy may also be useful for subjects with perinatal brain injury.

6.8 Conclusion

UC-MSCs have recently attracted considerable attention due to their convenient and minimally invasive collection, undifferentiated state, multilineage potential, immunosuppressive capacity, and clinical efficacy.

Clinical trials of UC-MSC administration for neurological disorders are ongoing, and improvements are expected in these patients. Based on these fundamental experiments and clinical studies, perinatal brain injuries will be also treated with UC-MSCs in the near future.

References

1. Gnecchi M, Melo LG. Bone marrow-derived mesenchymal stem cells: isolation, expansion, characterization, viral transduction, and production of conditioned medium. Methods Mol Biol. 2009;482:281–94.
2. Bieback K, Kluter H. Mesenchymal stromal cells from umbilical cord blood. Curr Stem Cell Res Ther. 2007;2(4):310–23.
3. Gruber HE, Deepe R, Hoelscher GL, Ingram JA, Norton HJ, Scannell B, et al. Human adipose-derived mesenchymal stem cells: direction to a phenotype sharing similarities with the disc, gene expression profiling, and coculture with human annulus cells. Tissue Eng Part A. 2010;16(9):2843–60.

4. In 't Anker PS, Scherjon SA, Kleijburg-van der Keur C, de Groot-Swings GM, Claas FH, Fibbe WE, et al. Isolation of mesenchymal stem cells of fetal or maternal origin from human placenta. Stem Cells. 2004;22(7):1338–45.
5. Romanov YA, Svintsitskaya VA, Smirnov VN. Searching for alternative sources of postnatal human mesenchymal stem cells: candidate MSC-like cells from umbilical cord. Stem Cells. 2003;21(1):105–10.
6. McElreavey KD, Irvine AI, Ennis KT, McLean WH. Isolation, culture and characterisation of fibroblast-like cells derived from the Wharton's jelly portion of human umbilical cord. Biochem Soc Trans. 1991;19(1):29S.
7. He H, Nagamura-Inoue T, Takahashi A, Mori Y, Yamamoto Y, Shimazu T, et al. Immunosuppressive properties of Wharton's jelly-derived mesenchymal stromal cells in vitro. International journal of hematology. 2015;102(3):368–78.
8. Nagamura-Inoue T, He H. Umbilical cord-derived mesenchymal stem cells: their advantages and potential clinical utility. World J Stem Cells. 2014;6(2):195–202.
9. Ahn SY, Chang YS, Park WS. Mesenchymal stem cells transplantation for neuroprotection in preterm infants with severe intraventricular hemorrhage. Korean J Pediatr. 2014;57(6):251–6.
10. Majore I, Moretti P, Stahl F, Hass R, Kasper C. Growth and differentiation properties of mesenchymal stromal cell populations derived from whole human umbilical cord. Stem Cell Rev. 2011;7(1):17–31.
11. Marmotti A, Mattia S, Bruzzone M, Buttiglieri S, Risso A, Bonasia DE, et al. Minced umbilical cord fragments as a source of cells for orthopaedic tissue engineering: an in vitro study. Stem Cells Int. 2012;2012:326813.
12. Mori Y, Ohshimo J, Shimazu T, He H, Takahashi A, Yamamoto Y, et al. Improved explant method to isolate umbilical cord-derived mesenchymal stem cells and their immunosuppressive properties. Tissue Eng Part C Methods. 2015;21(4):367–72.
13. Kikuchi-Taura A, Taguchi A, Kanda T, Inoue T, Kasahara Y, Hirose H, et al. Human umbilical cord provides a significant source of unexpanded mesenchymal stromal cells. Cytotherapy. 2012;14(4):441–50.
14. Salehinejad P, Alitheen NB, Ali AM, Omar AR, Mohit M, Janzamin E, et al. Comparison of different methods for the isolation of mesenchymal stem cells from human umbilical cord Wharton's jelly. In Vitro Cell Dev Biol Anim. 2012;48(2):75–83.
15. Ennis J, Gotherstrom C, Le Blanc K, Davies JE. In vitro immunologic properties of human umbilical cord perivascular cells. Cytotherapy. 2008;10(2):174–81.
16. Leroux P, Omouendze PL, Roy V, Dourmap N, Gonzalez BJ, Brasse-Lagnel C, et al. Age-dependent neonatal intracerebral hemorrhage in plasminogen activator inhibitor 1 knockout mice. J Neuropathol Exp Neurol. 2014;73(5):387–402.
17. Shimazu T. Serum- and xeno-free cryopreservation of human umbilical cord tissue as mesenchymal stromal cell source. Cytotherapy. 2015;17(5):593–600.
18. Dominici M, Le Blanc K, Mueller I, Slaper-Cortenbach I, Marini F, Krause D, et al. Minimal criteria for defining multipotent mesenchymal stromal cells. The International Society for Cellular Therapy position statement. Cytotherapy. 2006;8(4):315–7.
19. Horwitz EM, Le Blanc K, Dominici M, Mueller I, Slaper-Cortenbach I, Marini FC, et al. Clarification of the nomenclature for MSC: the International Society for Cellular Therapy position statement. Cytotherapy. 2005;7(5):393–5.
20. Mennan C, Wright K, Bhattacharjee A, Balain B, Richardson J, Roberts S. Isolation and characterisation of mesenchymal stem cells from different regions of the human umbilical cord. BioMed Res Int. 2013;2013:1–8.
21. He H, Nagamura-Inoue T, Tsunoda H, Yuzawa M, Yamamoto Y, Yorozu P, et al. Stage-specific embryonic antigen 4 in Wharton's jellyderived mesenchymal stem cells is not a marker for proliferation and multipotency. Tissue engineering Part A. 2014;20(7–8):1314–24.
22. Guo L, Zhou Y, Wang S, Wu Y. Epigenetic changes of mesenchymal stem cells in three-dimensional (3D) spheroids. J Cell Mol Med. 2014;18(10):2009–19.
23. Krampera M, Glennie S, Dyson J, Scott D, Laylor R, Simpson E, et al. Bone marrow mesenchymal stem cells inhibit the response of naive and memory antigen-specific T cells to their cognate peptide. Blood. 2003;101(9):3722–9.

24. Weiss ML, Anderson C, Medicetty S, Seshareddy KB, Weiss RJ, VanderWerff I, et al. Immune properties of human umbilical cord Wharton's jelly-derived cells. Stem Cells. 2008;26(11):2865–74.
25. English K, Barry FP, Mahon BP. Murine mesenchymal stem cells suppress dendritic cell migration, maturation and antigen presentation. Immunol Lett. 2008;115(1):50–8.
26. Spaggiari GM, Capobianco A, Abdelrazik H, Becchetti F, Mingari MC, Moretta L. Mesenchymal stem cells inhibit natural killer-cell proliferation, cytotoxicity, and cytokine production: role of indoleamine 2,3-dioxygenase and prostaglandin E2. Blood. 2008;111(3):1327–33.
27. Asari S, Itakura S, Ferreri K, Liu CP, Kuroda Y, Kandeel F, et al. Mesenchymal stem cells suppress B-cell terminal differentiation. Exp Hematol. 2009;37(5):604–15.
28. Magatti M, De Munari S, Vertua E, Gibelli L, Wengler GS, Parolini O. Human amnion mesenchyme harbors cells with allogeneic T-cell suppression and stimulation capabilities. Stem Cells. 2008;26(1):182–92.
29. Seshareddy K, Troyer D, Weiss ML. Method to isolate mesenchymal-like cells from Wharton's Jelly of umbilical cord. Methods Cell Biol. 2008;86:101–19.
30. Zhou C, Yang B, Tian Y, Jiao H, Zheng W, Wang J, et al. Immunomodulatory effect of human umbilical cord Wharton's jelly-derived mesenchymal stem cells on lymphocytes. Cell Immunol. 2011;272(1):33–8.
31. Valencic E, Piscianz E, Andolina M, Ventura A, Tommasini A. The immunosuppressive effect of Wharton's jelly stromal cells depends on the timing of their licensing and on lymphocyte activation. Cytotherapy. 2010;12(2):154–60.
32. Deuse T, Stubbendorff M, Tang-Quan K, Phillips N, Kay MA, Eiermann T, et al. Immunogenicity and immunomodulatory properties of umbilical cord lining mesenchymal stem cells. Cell Transplant. 2011;20(5):655–67.
33. Batsali AK, Kastrinaki MC, Papadaki HA, Pontikoglou C. Mesenchymal stem cells derived from Wharton's Jelly of the umbilical cord: biological properties and emerging clinical applications. Curr Stem Cell Res Ther. 2013;8(2):144–55.
34. Han X, Yang Q, Lin L, Xu C, Zheng C, Chen X, et al. Interleukin-17 enhances immunosuppression by mesenchymal stem cells. Cell Death Differ. 2014;21(11):1758–68.
35. Wang HS, Hung SC, Peng ST, Huang CC, Wei HM, Guo YJ, et al. Mesenchymal stem cells in the Wharton's jelly of the human umbilical cord. Stem Cells. 2004;22(7):1330–7.
36. Karahuseyinoglu S, Cinar O, Kilic E, Kara F, Akay GG, Demiralp DO, et al. Biology of stem cells in human umbilical cord stroma: in situ and in vitro surveys. Stem Cells. 2007;25(2):319–31.
37. Huang YC, Parolini O, La Rocca G, Deng L. Umbilical cord versus bone marrow-derived mesenchymal stromal cells. Stem Cells Dev. 2012;21(15):2900–3.
38. Fong CY, Gauthaman K, Cheyyatraivendran S, Lin HD, Biswas A, Bongso A. Human umbilical cord Wharton's jelly stem cells and its conditioned medium support hematopoietic stem cell expansion ex vivo. J Cell Biochem. 2012;113(2):658–68.
39. Fong CY, Subramanian A, Gauthaman K, Venugopal J, Biswas A, Ramakrishna S, et al. Human umbilical cord Wharton's jelly stem cells undergo enhanced chondrogenic differentiation when grown on nanofibrous scaffolds and in a sequential two-stage culture medium environment. Stem Cell Rev. 2012;8(1):195–209.
40. Hsieh JY, Fu YS, Chang SJ, Tsuang YH, Wang HW. Functional module analysis reveals differential osteogenic and stemness potentials in human mesenchymal stem cells from bone marrow and Wharton's jelly of umbilical cord. Stem Cells Dev. 2010;19(12):1895–910.
41. Zeddou M, Relic B, Malaise O, Charlier E, Desoroux A, Beguin Y, et al. Differential signalling through ALK-1 and ALK-5 regulates leptin expression in mesenchymal stem cells. Stem Cells Dev. 2012;21(11):1948–55.
42. Leite C, Silva NT, Mendes S, Ribeiro A, de Faria JP, Lourenco T, et al. Differentiation of human umbilical cord matrix mesenchymal stem cells into neural-like progenitor cells and maturation into an oligodendroglial-like lineage. PLoS One. 2014;9(10):e111059.
43. Scuteri A, Miloso M, Foudah D, Orciani M, Cavaletti G, Tredici G. Mesenchymal stem cells neuronal differentiation ability: a real perspective for nervous system repair? Curr Stem Cell Res Ther. 2011;6(2):82–92.

44. Hsieh JY, Wang HW, Chang SJ, Liao KH, Lee IH, Lin WS, et al. Mesenchymal stem cells from human umbilical cord express preferentially secreted factors related to neuroprotection, neurogenesis, and angiogenesis. PLoS One. 2013;8(8):e72604.
45. Mukai T, Nagamura-Inoue T, Shimazu T, Mori Y, Takahashi A, Tsunoda H, et al. Neurosphere formation enhances the neurogenic differentiation potential and migratory ability of umbilical cord-mesenchymal stromal cells. Cytotherapy. 2016;18(2):229–41.
46. Takenouchi T, Iwata O, Nabetani M, Tamura M. Therapeutic hypothermia for neonatal encephalopathy: JSPNM & MHLW Japan working group practice guidelines consensus statement from the working group on therapeutic hypothermia for neonatal encephalopathy, Ministry of Health, labor and welfare (MHLW), Japan, and Japan Society for Perinatal and Neonatal Medicine (JSPNM). Brain Dev. 2012;34(2):165–70.
47. van Velthoven CT, Kavelaars A, van Bel F, Heijnen CJ. Mesenchymal stem cell treatment after neonatal hypoxic-ischemic brain injury improves behavioral outcome and induces neuronal and oligodendrocyte regeneration. Brain Behav Immun. 2010;24(3):387–93.
48. Jellema RK, Wolfs TG, Lima Passos V, Zwanenburg A, Ophelders DR, Kuypers E, et al. Mesenchymal stem cells induce T-cell tolerance and protect the preterm brain after global hypoxia-ischemia. PLoS One. 2013;8(8):e73031.
49. Ding DC, Shyu WC, Chiang MF, Lin SZ, Chang YC, Wang HJ, et al. Enhancement of neuroplasticity through upregulation of beta1-integrin in human umbilical cord-derived stromal cell implanted stroke model. Neurobiol Dis. 2007;27(3):339–53.
50. Zhu LH, Bai X, Zhang N, Wang SY, Li W, Jiang L. Improvement of human umbilical cord mesenchymal stem cell transplantation on glial cell and behavioral function in a neonatal model of periventricular white matter damage. Brain Res. 2014;1563:13–21.
51. Cheng Q, Zhang Z, Zhang S, Yang H, Zhang X, Pan J, et al. Human umbilical cord mesenchymal stem cells protect against ischemic brain injury in mouse by regulating peripheral immunoinflammation. Brain Res. 2015;1594:293–304.
52. Mukai T, Mori Y, Shimazu T, Takahashi A, Tsunoda H, Yamaguchi S, et al. Intravenous injection of umbilical cord-derived mesenchymal stromal cells attenuates reactive gliosis and hypomyelination in a neonatal intraventricular hemorrhage model. Neuroscience. 2017; 355:175–87.
53. Geffner LF, Santacruz P, Izurieta M, Flor L, Maldonado B, Auad AH, et al. Administration of autologous bone marrow stem cells into spinal cord injury patients via multiple routes is safe and improves their quality of life: comprehensive case studies. Cell Transplant. 2008;17(12):1277–93.
54. Sykova E, Homola A, Mazanec R, Lachmann H, Konradova SL, Kobylka P, et al. Autologous bone marrow transplantation in patients with subacute and chronic spinal cord injury. Cell Transplant. 2006;15(8–9):675–87.
55. Bang OY, Lee JS, Lee PH, Lee G. Autologous mesenchymal stem cell transplantation in stroke patients. Ann Neurol. 2005;57(6):874–82.
56. Wang L, Wang Q, Zhang XM. Progress on bone marrow mesenchymal stem cells transplantation for spinal cord injury. China J Orthop Traumatol. 2014;27(5):437–40.
57. Dongmei H, Jing L, Mei X, Ling Z, Hongmin Y, Zhidong W, et al. Clinical analysis of the treatment of spinocerebellar ataxia and multiple system atrophy-cerebellar type with umbilical cord mesenchymal stromal cells. Cytotherapy. 2011;13(8):913–7.
58. Jin JL, Liu Z, Lu ZJ, Guan DN, Wang C, Chen ZB, et al. Safety and efficacy of umbilical cord mesenchymal stem cell therapy in hereditary spinocerebellar ataxia. Curr Neurovasc Res. 2013;10(1):11–20.
59. Wang S, Cheng H, Dai G, Wang X, Hua R, Liu X, et al. Umbilical cord mesenchymal stem cell transplantation significantly improves neurological function in patients with sequelae of traumatic brain injury. Brain Res. 2013;1532:76–84.
60. Wang X, Hu H, Hua R, Yang J, Zheng P, Niu X, et al. Effect of umbilical cord mesenchymal stromal cells on motor functions of identical twins with cerebral palsy: pilot study on the correlation of efficacy and hereditary factors. Cytotherapy. 2015;17(2):224–31.
61. Nagamura-Inoue T, Mukai T. Umbilical cord is a rich source of mesenchymal stromal cells for cell therapy. Curr Stem Cell Res Ther. 2016;11(8):634–42.

Chapter 7
Other Tissues-Derived Mesenchymal Stem Cells for Perinatal Brain Injury

Yoshiaki Sato

Abstract Cell-based treatments are emerging as a potential therapy for perinatal brain injury. Neural stem/progenitor cells (NSPCs) have been studied primarily in preclinical models of HIE. However, despite their neural commitment, ethical concerns hinder the use of postmortem human brains as a source of NSPCs in future clinical applications. Furthermore, intracerebral administration is an invasive procedure.

Stem cells originating from nonneural tissues can provide an approach that avoids these limitations. The stem cells from nonneural tissues, such as umbilical cord blood cells (UCBCs) and mesenchymal stem cells (MSCs), have a broad potential for differentiation, into mesodermal, endodermal, and ectodermal lineages.

UCBCs have an advantage in that we can perform autologous transplantation if we get them at birth; however, it is conceivable that we might often encounter difficulties collecting UCBCs in emergency situations.

MSCs can be used as alternative cells for the treatment of perinatal HIE because we can use allogeneic MSCs. In this chapter, I describe preclinical studies with various origins of MSCs as well as clinical studies.

Keywords Mesenchymal stem cell · Adipose tissue · Dedifferentiated fat cell

7.1 Introduction

Cell-based treatments are emerging as a potential therapy for perinatal brain injury. Various kinds of stem cells with both fetal and adult origins may be promising for the treatment of neonatal ischemic brain injury via their potential for protecting host

Y. Sato, M.D., Ph.D.
Division of Neonatology, Center for Maternal-Neonatal Care,
Nagoya University Hospital, Nagoya, Japan
e-mail: yoshiaki@med.nagoya-u.ac.jp

© Springer Nature Singapore Pte Ltd. 2018

H. Shintaku et al. (eds.), *Cell Therapy for Perinatal Brain Injury*,
https://doi.org/10.1007/978-981-10-1412-3_7

cells, promoting their growth and differentiation, and regulating the host immune response [1, 2]. As described in Chap. 4, neural stem/progenitor cells (NSPCs) have been studied primarily in preclinical models of HIE. After their cortical transplantation or intraventricular injection, they can migrate, integrate, and differentiate into neurons and oligodendrocytes in perinatal hypoxic-ischemic (HI) models [3–5]. However, despite their neural commitment, ethical concerns hinder the use of postmortem human brains as a source of NSPCs in future clinical applications. Furthermore, intracerebral administration is an invasive procedure, and the injected cells themselves may lead to gliotic changes in the host brain [6], thereby necessitating more detailed examinations to ensure the safety of the procedure.

Stem cells originating from nonneural tissues can provide an approach that avoids these limitations. In contrast to the initial belief that they are restricted to their tissue of origin, the stem cells from nonneural tissues, such as umbilical cord blood cells (UCBCs) and mesenchymal stem cells (MSCs), have a broad potential for differentiation, into mesodermal, endodermal, and ectodermal lineages.

UCBCs have an advantage in that we can perform autologous transplantation if we get them at birth, and clinical trials using UCBCs for perinatal HI have already begun (see Chap. 1). However, it is conceivable that we might often encounter difficulties collecting UCBCs in emergency situations, such as in cases of precipitous delivery. Therefore, we should develop an alternative treatment for infants who miss the opportunity for UCBC therapy. Alternative treatments should be ones in which we can perform allogenic transplantation or ones using cells we collect after admission.

MSCs have intrinsic anti-inflammatory and immunomodulatory properties. In addition, these have little or zero major histocompatibility class II antigen expression [7]. Although allogeneic MSCs administered can induce antidonor responses to some degree [8], allogeneic and autologous MSCs were found to be similarly effective in some disease models [9]; further, in related perinatal HI, allotransplantation or even xenotransplantation demonstrated treatment effect [10]. I expect that MSCs can be used as alternative cells for the treatment of perinatal HIE.

7.2 Preclinical Studies with Various Origins of MSCs for Perinatal HI

MSCs can be isolated from various tissues, including bone marrow, adipose tissue, placental tissue, umbilical cord, and dental pulp. In this chapter, I describe preclinical studies with various origins of MSCs (except one derived from umbilical cord, which is reviewed in Chap. 6).

Among various MSCs, bone marrow-derived MSCs seem to be the most common, and more preclinical studies have already emerged. Yasuhara et al. [11] published the first report using MSCs for perinatal HI. They injected cells into the hippocampus and showed motor deficits associated with HI injury. The same group investigated differences between intravenous and intracerebral injections [12]. They showed that intravenous injection with the same number of cells exerted the same degree of treatment effect as intracerebral injection. Intravenous injection is potentially more practical and less invasive in clinical application.

Several other groups showed the treatment effect of the bone marrow-derived MSCs with intracranial injection. Velthoven et al. reported the effect in several publications [13–16]; cerebral injection of MSCs 3 days after the insult improved behavioral outcomes and induced neuronal and oligodendrocyte regeneration [13]. Moreover, repeated MSC treatment had distinct effects on formation and maturation of new neurons and oligodendrocytes, which led to restoration of damaged areas, corticospinal motor tract activity, and sensorimotor function [14]. In another publication from the same group, it was shown that at 3 days after injection, only 22% of transplanted MSCs were detectable and 18 days after the last administration, barely 1% was detectable, indicating that engraftment of MSCs is not likely the underlying mechanism of the efficient regenerative process [15]. Additionally, they showed that the expression of genes induced by MCS injection was related to proliferation, survival, or growth.

Gu et al. performed intracerebroventricular injections of MSCs after the HI insult. They showed MSCs decrease apoptosis and improve learning-memory function induced by the HI insult and decrease IL-10 release via the TLR2/NFκB pathway [17]; additionally, they showed the endogenous IL-6 of MSCs mediated the neuroprotective effect with anti-apoptosis of injured astrocytes [18].

Lee et al. administered MSCs via intracardiac injection [19]. Intracardiac injection seems to be a difficult procedure and is not practical clinically. However, in neonatal medicine, immediately after birth, when infants present with perinatal HI, the umbilical artery can be catheterized up into the left ventricle of the heart. Therefore, MSCs can be injected intracardially through the umbilical artery catheter. Intracardiac injection can lead to deliver more MSCs to the injured brain, whereas most MSCs are trapped in the spleen, lung, or liver when injected intravenously.

Recently, another unique route for the administration of cells into the brain has emerged—intranasal [20]. Intracranial injections were often used in preclinical studies, but in clinical situations, there are challenges with direct injection into the brain. For severely asphyxiated neonates, not only the neurologic but also general health condition is often poor. Therefore, these patients cannot be transported to computed tomography (CT), which is required for proper injection placement. Furthermore, such neonates are more likely to be hypocoagulable, so injection into the brain is more likely to induce intracranial bleeding. Intravenous administration is also used in many preclinical studies and has shown treatment effect, but many of the intravenously injected cells can be trapped in other organs, including the lung as described above. Intravenous injection of a greater number of cells potentially risks embolism to the lung. Conversely, MSCs can cross the cribriform plate when administered intranasally and migrated throughout the brain using the rostral migratory stream [21].

With this unique route, Heijnen's group in the Netherlands has been performing several preclinical studies. Intranasal MSC treatment significantly improved sensorimotor function in the cylinder rearing test and decreased gray and white matter loss [20]. In addition to sensorimotor function, intranasal MSC treatment after HI improves cognitive function [22]. MSCs reached the lesion site within 2 h after intranasal administration. The number of MSCs at the lesion site peaks at 12 h after administration and decreases gradually after that. The MSCs promoted neurogenesis and a decrease in reactive astrocytes and microglia, as well as polarization of microglia toward the M2 phenotype [23]. Furthermore, the long-term efficacy and safety up to 14 months in the mouse was shown [24]. In addition, there was successful treatment effect using both rodent as well as human MSCs [10].

As described in other Chaps. 1, 5, and 6, umbilical cord/umbilical cord blood is used widely as a stem cell source. Umbilical cord blood (UCB)-derived MSCs have also been studied as a treatment for perinatal brain injury. Park et al. evaluated the effect of combination therapy with hypothermia and UCB-derived MSCs, and all of the abnormalities observed in histological or functional analyses in severe HIE demonstrated greater improvement after combined treatment with hypothermia and MSC transplantation than with either therapy alone [25]. The same group evaluated the treatment effect on severe intraventricular hemorrhage. Intraventricular transplantation of umbilical cord blood-derived MSCs prevented posthemorrhagic hydrocephalus development and attenuated impairment on behavioral tests [26]; even with intravenous injection, the effect was almost identical [27].

Recently, adipose tissue has emerged as an appealing source of stem cells. Adipose tissue can be an ideal stem cell source because it is (1) abundant, (2) easily accessible via minimally invasive procedures (liposuction aspiration or needle biopsy), and (3) has low immunogenicity, which facilitates allogeneic as well as autologous transplantations [28]. MSCs in the stromal vascular fraction (SVF) of the adipose tissue are called "adipose-derived stem/stromal cells (ASCs)" and exhibit multipotency differentiating along the adipocyte, chondrocyte, myocyte, neuronal, and osteoblast lineages [29]. Park et al. intracerebroventricularly transplanted human ASCs into neonatal rats treated with hypoxia-ischemia-lipopolysaccharide and showed a treatment effect histologically and behaviorally [30].

In contrast with SVF, the predominant cell type in adipose tissue is mature adipocytes. The simple ceiling culture technique makes them dedifferentiate into fibroblast-like cells with a high proliferative capacity [31]. The newly established cell line, called dedifferentiated fat (DFAT) cells, exhibits characteristics comparable to ASCs in SVF [32, 33]. DFAT cells represent a more homogeneous cell group, which yields cultures with higher purity compared to ASCs. In prolonged cultures, DFAT can retain their expansion capacity and phenotype better than ASCs, where the immunophenotype of the latter changed gradually through different passages [34].

We evaluated whether the outcome of HIE can be improved by DFAT cell treatment. DFAT cells injected intravenously suppressed the apoptosis, microglial activation, and oxidative stress, induced by HI. In addition, no difference was confirmed between the DFAT and sham groups in motor function according to the rotarod treadmill and cylinder test, whereas there was a significant difference in the vehicle group. According to in vitro experiments, the cell death rates of neurons treated in the conditioned medium (CM) prepared from cultured DFAT cells were significantly lower than those in the controls. In the DFAT-CM, several neurotrophic factors (IGF-1, NGF, NT3) were detected, and these factors were increased in the ipsilateral brain after injection of DFAT. Our results indicate that intravenous injection with DFAT cells is effective for ameliorating HI brain injury, possibly via paracrine effects.

Another unique stem source is dental pulp stem cells. The dental pulp is readily obtained, for example, via extracted third molars or exfoliated deciduous teeth. These stem cells were identified to be a proliferative population of clonogenic cells and differentiate into a variety of cell types: neural cells, adipocytes, odontoblasts, osteoblasts, and endothelial cells. In addition, these are harvestable from primary teeth or third molars as medical waste, leading to very few ethical problems for usage. Moreover, the stem cells are derived from the neural crest with undifferentiated system markers, showing differentiation potential-like neural stem cells.

Yamagata et al. investigated the therapeutic effects of stem cells from human exfoliated deciduous teeth (SHED). They injected SHED into the injured brain and showed remarkable neurological and pathophysiological recovery. Notably, the intracerebral administration of SHED-CM also exerts a significantly treatment effect [35]. Fang et al. used the stem cells from extracted third molars. They injected the cells into the left lateral ventricle in injured brain and showed a treatment effect behaviorally and histologically [36].

7.3 Clinical Studies for Perinatal Brain Injury with MSCs

According to ClinicalTrial.gov, there have been clinical trials with MSCs only for intraventricular hemorrhage to date. In these studies, Pneumostem® (human umbilical cord blood-derived MSCs) was used, which was used for clinical trials in bronchopulmonary dysplasia (BPD). A Phase 1 study (NCT02274428) has already been completed by Samsung Medical Center in Korea, and a Phase 2 study (NCT02890953) is ongoing. The inclusion criteria in this study are intraventricular hemorrhage grades 3–4, within postnatal day 28, and gestational age: 23–<34 weeks. And death or requirement of shunt operation will be the primary outcome between Pneumostem® and normal saline groups.

7.4 Conclusions

In this chapter, preclinical and clinical studies with MSCs for perinatal HI were reviewed. Although only a few clinical trials have been started, many preclinical trial with animals have shown promising treatment effect. As described in the introduction section, to apply the cell therapy to many HIE patients, allogenic transplantation or cells which we can collect after admission should be needed. MSCs are expected to be ideal stem cells for the treatment of perinatal HIE.

References

1. Bennet L, Tan S, Van den Heuij L, Derrick M, Groenendaal F, van Bel F, et al. Cell therapy for neonatal hypoxia-ischemia and cerebral palsy. Ann Neurol. 2012;71(5):589–600. https://doi.org/10.1002/ana.22670.
2. Titomanlio L, Kavelaars A, Dalous J, Mani S, El Ghouzzi V, Heijnen C, et al. Stem cell therapy for neonatal brain injury: perspectives and challenges. Ann Neurol. 2011;70(5):698–712. https://doi.org/10.1002/ana.22518.
3. Felling RJ, Snyder MJ, Romanko MJ, Rothstein RP, Ziegler AN, Yang Z, et al. Neural stem/progenitor cells participate in the regenerative response to perinatal hypoxia/ischemia. J Neurosci. 2006;26(16):4359–69. https://doi.org/10.1523/JNEUROSCI.1898-05.2006.
4. Sato Y, Nakanishi K, Hayakawa M, Kakizawa H, Saito A, Kuroda Y, et al. Reduction of brain injury in neonatal hypoxic-ischemic rats by intracerebroventricular injection of neural stem/progenitor cells together with chondroitinase ABC. Reprod Sci. 2008;15(6):613–20. https://doi.org/10.1177/1933719108317299.
5. Sato Y, Oohira A. Chondroitin sulfate, a major niche substance of neural stem cells, and cell transplantation therapy of neurodegeneration combined with niche modification. Curr Stem Cell Res Ther. 2009;4(3):200–9.
6. Sato Y, Shinjyo N, Sato M, Osato K, Zhu C, Pekna M, et al. Grafting of neural stem and progenitor cells to the hippocampus of young, irradiated mice causes gliosis and disrupts the granule cell layer. Cell Death Dis. 2013;4:e591. https://doi.org/10.1038/cddis.2013.92.
7. Le Blanc K, Pittenger M. Mesenchymal stem cells: progress toward promise. Cytotherapy. 2005;7(1):36–45. https://doi.org/10.1080/14653240510018118.
8. Zangi L, Margalit R, Reich-Zeliger S, Bachar-Lustig E, Beilhack A, Negrin R, et al. Direct imaging of immune rejection and memory induction by allogeneic mesenchymal stromal cells. Stem Cells. 2009;27(11):2865–74. https://doi.org/10.1002/stem.217.
9. van Velthoven CT, Kavelaars A, Heijnen CJ. Mesenchymal stem cells as a treatment for neonatal ischemic brain damage. Pediatr Res. 2012a;71(4 Pt 2):474–81. https://doi.org/10.1038/pr.2011.64.
10. Donega V, Nijboer CH, Braccioli L, Slaper-Cortenbach I, Kavelaars A, van Bel F, et al. Intranasal administration of human MSC for ischemic brain injury in the mouse: in vitro and in vivo neuroregenerative functions. PLoS One. 2014a;9(11):e112339. https://doi.org/10.1371/journal.pone.0112339.
11. Yasuhara T, Matsukawa N, Yu G, Xu L, Mays RW, Kovach J, et al. Behavioral and histological characterization of intrahippocampal grafts of human bone marrow-derived multipotent progenitor cells in neonatal rats with hypoxic-ischemic injury. Cell Transplant. 2006;15(3):231–8.
12. Yasuhara T, Hara K, Maki M, Mays RW, Deans RJ, Hess DC, et al. Intravenous grafts recapitulate the neurorestoration afforded by intracerebrally delivered multipotent adult progenitor cells in neonatal hypoxic-ischemic rats. J Cereb Blood Flow Metab. 2008;28(11):1804–10. https://doi.org/10.1038/jcbfm.2008.68.
13. van Velthoven CT, Kavelaars A, van Bel F, Heijnen CJ. Mesenchymal stem cell treatment after neonatal hypoxic-ischemic brain injury improves behavioral outcome and induces neuronal and oligodendrocyte regeneration. Brain Behav Immun. 2010a;24(3):387–93. https://doi.org/10.1016/j.bbi.2009.10.017.
14. van Velthoven CT, Kavelaars A, van Bel F, Heijnen CJ. Repeated mesenchymal stem cell treatment after neonatal hypoxia-ischemia has distinct effects on formation and maturation

of new neurons and oligodendrocytes leading to restoration of damage, corticospinal motor tract activity, and sensorimotor function. J Neurosci. 2010c;30(28):9603–11. https://doi.org/10.1523/JNEUROSCI.1835-10.2010.

15. van Velthoven CT, Kavelaars A, van Bel F, Heijnen CJ. Mesenchymal stem cell transplantation changes the gene expression profile of the neonatal ischemic brain. Brain Behav Immun. 2011;25(7):1342–8. https://doi.org/10.1016/j.bbi.2011.03.021.
16. van Velthoven CT, van de Looij Y, Kavelaars A, Zijlstra J, van Bel F, Huppi PS, et al. Mesenchymal stem cells restore cortical rewiring after neonatal ischemia in mice. Ann Neurol. 2012b;71(6):785–96. https://doi.org/10.1002/ana.23543.
17. Gu Y, Zhang Y, Bi Y, Liu J, Tan B, Gong M, et al. Mesenchymal stem cells suppress neuronal apoptosis and decrease IL-10 release via the TLR2/NFkappaB pathway in rats with hypoxic-ischemic brain damage. Mol Brain. 2015;8(1):65. https://doi.org/10.1186/s13041-015-0157-3.
18. Gu Y, He M, Zhou X, Liu J, Hou N, Bin T, et al. Endogenous IL-6 of mesenchymal stem cell improves behavioral outcome of hypoxic-ischemic brain damage neonatal rats by supressing apoptosis in astrocyte. Sci Rep. 2016;6:18587. https://doi.org/10.1038/srep18587.
19. Lee JA, Kim BI, Jo CH, Choi CW, Kim EK, Kim HS, et al. Mesenchymal stem-cell transplantation for hypoxic-ischemic brain injury in neonatal rat model. Pediatr Res. 2009;67(1):42–6. https://doi.org/10.1203/PDR.0b013e3181bf594b.
20. van Velthoven CT, Kavelaars A, van Bel F, Heijnen CJ. Nasal administration of stem cells: a promising novel route to treat neonatal ischemic brain damage. Pediatr Res. 2010b;68(5):419–22. https://doi.org/10.1203/PDR.0b013e3181f1c289.
21. Danielyan L, Schafer R, von Ameln-Mayerhofer A, Buadze M, Geisler J, Klopfer T, et al. Intranasal delivery of cells to the brain. Eur J Cell Biol. 2009;88(6):315–24. https://doi.org/10.1016/j.ejcb.2009.02.001.
22. Donega V, van Velthoven CT, Nijboer CH, van Bel F, Kas MJ, Kavelaars A, et al. Intranasal mesenchymal stem cell treatment for neonatal brain damage: long-term cognitive and sensorimotor improvement. PLoS One. 2013;8(1):e51253. https://doi.org/10.1371/journal.pone.0051253.
23. Donega V, Nijboer CH, van Tilborg G, Dijkhuizen RM, Kavelaars A, Heijnen CJ. Intranasally administered mesenchymal stem cells promote a regenerative niche for repair of neonatal ischemic brain injury. Exp Neurol. 2014b;261:53–64. https://doi.org/10.1016/j.expneurol.2014.06.009.
24. Donega V, Nijboer CH, van Velthoven CT, Youssef SA, de Bruin A, van Bel F, et al. Assessment of long-term safety and efficacy of intranasal mesenchymal stem cell treatment for neonatal brain injury in the mouse. Pediatr Res. 2015;78(5):520–6. https://doi.org/10.1038/pr.2015.145.
25. Park WS, Sung SI, Ahn SY, Yoo HS, Sung DK, Im GH, et al. Hypothermia augments neuroprotective activity of mesenchymal stem cells for neonatal hypoxic-ischemic encephalopathy. PLoS One. 2015;10(3):e0120893. https://doi.org/10.1371/journal.pone.0120893.
26. Ahn SY, Chang YS, Sung DK, Sung SI, Yoo HS, Lee JH, et al. Mesenchymal stem cells prevent hydrocephalus after severe intraventricular hemorrhage. Stroke. 2013;44(2):497–504. https://doi.org/10.1161/strokeaha.112.679092.
27. Ahn SY, Chang YS, Sung DK, Sung SI, Yoo HS, Im GH, et al. Optimal route for mesenchymal stem cells transplantation after severe intraventricular hemorrhage in newborn rats. PLoS One. 2015;10(7):e0132919. https://doi.org/10.1371/journal.pone.0132919.
28. Bunnell BA, Flaat M, Gagliardi C, Patel B, Ripoll C. Adipose-derived stem cells: isolation, expansion and differentiation. Methods. 2008;45(2):115–20. https://doi.org/10.1016/j.ymeth.2008.03.006.
29. Gimble J, Guilak F. Adipose-derived adult stem cells: isolation, characterization, and differentiation potential. Cytotherapy. 2003;5(5):362–9. https://doi.org/10.1080/14653240310003026.
30. Park D, Lee SH, Bae DK, Yang YH, Yang G, Kyung J, et al. Transplantation of human adipose tissue-derived Mesenchymal stem cells restores the neurobehavioral disorders of rats with neonatal hypoxic-ischemic encephalopathy. Cell Med. 2013;5(1):17–28. https://doi.org/10.3727/215517913x658936.

31. Sugihara H, Yonemitsu N, Miyabara S, Yun K. Primary cultures of unilocular fat cells: characteristics of growth in vitro and changes in differentiation properties. Differentiation. 1986;31(1):42–9.
32. Matsumoto T, Kano K, Kondo D, Fukuda N, Iribe Y, Tanaka N, et al. Mature adipocyte-derived dedifferentiated fat cells exhibit multilineage potential. J Cell Physiol. 2008;215(1):210–22. https://doi.org/10.1002/jcp.21304.
33. Yagi K, Kondo D, Okazaki Y, Kano K. A novel preadipocyte cell line established from mouse adult mature adipocytes. Biochem Biophys Res Commun. 2004;321(4):967–74. https://doi.org/10.1016/j.bbrc.2004.07.055.
34. Shen JF, Sugawara A, Yamashita J, Ogura H, Sato S. Dedifferentiated fat cells: an alternative source of adult multipotent cells from the adipose tissues. Int J Oral Sci. 2011;3(3):117–24. https://doi.org/10.4248/IJOS11044.
35. Yamagata M, Yamamoto A, Kako E, Kaneko N, Matsubara K, Sakai K, et al. Human dental pulp-derived stem cells protect against hypoxic-ischemic brain injury in neonatal mice. Stroke. 2013;44(2):551–4. https://doi.org/10.1161/STROKEAHA.112.676759.
36. Fang CZ, Yang YJ, Wang QH, Yao Y, Zhang XY, He XH. Intraventricular injection of human dental pulp stem cells improves hypoxic-ischemic brain damage in neonatal rats. PLoS One. 2013;8(6):e66748. https://doi.org/10.1371/journal.pone.0066748.

Chapter 8
CD34$^+$ Cell in Cord Blood and Neonates

Takashi Hamazaki and Haruo Shintaku

Abstract CD34 surface antigen has been extensively used as a marker for hematopoietic stem cells in adult bone marrow. Cord blood contains high number of hematopoietic and non-hematopoietic stem/progenitor cells. This chapter focuses on recent progresses in stem cell biology on cord blood cells. During embryonic development, expression of CD34 is tightly regulated in a spatial and temporal manner. Subpopulations of CD34$^+$ cells in cord blood have been characterized by their functional potency. CD133 positivity and aldehyde dehydrogenase activity are well overlapped to show higher regenerative potentials in CD34$^+$ cells. Proportion of CD34$^+$ cells tends to be higher in cord blood from preterm baby. The higher number of circulating CD34$^+$ cells in neonate has been found to be linked to the lower risk of prematurity-related complications. Further mechanistic studies will be required to reveal the role of circulating CD34$^+$ cells in neonate.

Keywords Cord blood · CD34 · Neonate · Hematopoietic stem cell

8.1 Introduction

In 1956, the first bone marrow transplantation was successfully performed to treat leukemia patient. Since then, biology of hematopoietic stem cells rapidly advanced and revealed that a small fraction of cells (hematopoietic stem cells) in bone marrow from donor engrafted and reconstituted the whole hematopoietic system in the recipient. The cells expressing CD34 antigen on their surface are capable to form robust colony in vitro and sufficient to reconstitute hematopoietic system when they are transplanted into myeloablative patients. CD34$^+$ cells in bone marrow, peripheral blood stem cells, and cord blood have been widely recognized as hematopoietic stem cells. The dosages of CD34$^+$ cells in transplanted cells are correlated with their engraftment outcomes. Therefore, laboratory test for enumeration of CD34$^+$ became

T. Hamazaki, M.D., Ph.D. (✉) • H. Shintaku, M.D., Ph.D.
Department of Pediatrics, Graduate School of Medicine, Osaka City University, Osaka, Japan
e-mail: hammer@med.osaka-cu.ac.jp

© Springer Nature Singapore Pte Ltd. 2018
H. Shintaku et al. (eds.), *Cell Therapy for Perinatal Brain Injury*,
https://doi.org/10.1007/978-981-10-1412-3_8

routine to evaluate quality of stem cells in transplantation practice. Organizations such as the European Group for Blood and Marrow Transplantation (EBMT) and International Society of Hematotherapy and Graft Engineering (ISHAGE) made great efforts to set analytical standard [1]. Although the minimum number of CD34$^+$ cells required for engraftment has not been firmly established, use of a minimum of 2×10^6 CD34$^+$ cells/kg is recommended for hematopoietic stem cell transplantation. In cases of cord blood cell transplantation, engraftment could be established more than 1 log lower CD34$^+$ cells suggesting higher reconstitution potentials of CD34$^+$ cells of cord blood [2].

8.2 Ontogeny of CD34$^+$ Cells During Pregnancy

Human hematopoiesis begins in the yolk sac (YS), called primitive hematopoiesis. In the YS, CD34 expression can be detected in endothelial cells derived from extra-embryonic mesoderm at 23 days of gestation. The YS generates primarily nucleated primitive erythroblasts to establish circulation. Then definitive hematopoiesis takes place in the ventral side of the aortic endothelium between the 27 and 40 days of gestation. The site is considered as the presumptive aorta-gonad-mesonephros (AGM) region. CD34$^+$ cell clusters can be found adjacent to this region [3]. The origin of this CD34$^+$ hematopoietic stem cells is still under debate whether they are from hematogenic endothelial cells or bi-potent hemangioblasts that give rise to both hematopoietic and endothelial cells [4]. The CD34$^+$ hematopoietic stem cells circulate in embryo and colonized into fetal liver after 30 days of gestation. The fetal liver turns into major site of hematopoiesis during embryogenesis [5]. Ultimately, the bone marrow also becomes the site of hematopoiesis at midgestation [6]. Based on recent comparative studies on cord blood between preterm and term baby, quantity and functional property of circulating CD34$^+$ cells in fetus seem to be dynamically changing until birth (see detail at Sect. 8.4 below). After birth, circulating CD34$^+$ cells rapidly decrease and bone marrow becomes a major site of hematopoiesis during the lifetime.

8.3 Subpopulation of CD34$^+$ Cells in Cord Blood

Despite the extensive use of CD34 analysis in transplantation medicine, biological function of CD34 protein remains enigmatic. CD34 antigen is a type of glycoprotein called sialomucin. Primary function of CD34 protein is postulated to regulate cell-to-cell adhesion [7]. Knockout studies on CD34 gene in mice showed only mild defects on hematopoiesis suggesting redundancy in their function [8, 9].

CD34$^+$ cells are containing various cell types rather than a uniform cell population. Moreover, the subset of CD34$^+$ cells varies depending on the source of hematopoietic stem cells: bone marrow, peripheral blood stem cells, and cord blood.

Research efforts have been made to identify long-term repopulating cells that are enriched in CD34^{+} cells. Functional assay to test whether certain subsets of cells can repopulate in nonobese diabetic/severe combined immunodeficiency (NOD/SCID) mice has been developed and widely accepted. These SCID-repopulating cells (SRCs) are considered as primitive hematopoietic stem cell to have higher engraftment potential. In bone marrow and cord blood, SRCs were enriched in CD34^{+}CD38$^{low/-}$ fraction, and no SRCs were found in CD34^{+}CD38^{high} subpopulation [10].

CD133 antigen also known as prominin-1 is a glycoprotein and expressed in wide spectrum of tissue-specific stem cells including hematopoietic stem cells, endothelial cells, or even brain tumors. The CD133^{+} cells in brain tumor are thought to be a cancer stem cell population, which can repopulate in immunodeficiency animals and is resistant to chemotherapeutic agents [11]. In cord blood, CD133^{+} cells can be found in both CD34^{+} and CD34^{-} cell fractions. Of interest, CD133^{+}cells from either the CD34^{+} or CD34^{-} fraction contain SRCs indicating long-term repopulating hematopoietic potentials [12]. Additionally CD133^{+}VEGFR-3^{+} cells in CD34^{+} fraction from fetal liver and bone marrow have shown to have a potential for lymphatic/vascular endothelial stem/precursor cells [13]. Majority of CD133^{+} cells in cord blood are expressing CD34 and vasculogenic functionality in ischemic animal models [14].

Instead of subtyping based on surface antigens, there are other ways to functionally subgrouping the potent stem cells. Measurement of aldehyde dehydrogenase (ALDH) activity has been proven to identify stem cell fraction in various normal and cancerous tissues [15, 16]. One fourth of CD34^{+} cells and two thirds of CD133^{+} cells from cord blood were also ALDH activity. CD34^{+} cells with high ALDH activity showed better long-term engraftment [17].

8.4 CD34^{+} Cells from Preterm vs. Term Neonate

Several studies have established whether quantitative and/or qualitative differences exist between cord blood collected from term and preterm neonates. There are large amounts of data available from public cord blood banking [18–21]. Table 8.1 summarizes the factors associated with the concentration of CD34^{+} cells in cord blood. Proportion of CD34^{+} cells tended to be higher in younger gestational age (34–37 weeks) than older (38 weeks or later) [21]. This tendency was also found in very preterm infants (24–32 weeks). Regarding differentiation potentials, in vitro clonogenic assay revealed that the number of erythrocyte burst-forming units (BFU-E) was significantly higher in preterm cord blood than in term cord blood. Isolated CD34^{+}CD133^{+}ALDH^{high} cells from preterm cord blood also exhibited higher clonogenic capacity than term cord blood cells suggesting that qualitative difference in subpopulation of CD34^{+} cells [22]. Based on the above studies, highly potent primitive hematopoietic stem cells were circulating during early gestational ages (24–36 weeks) and gradually homing into bone marrow niche toward late gestations.

Table 8.1 Factors associated with concentration of $CD34^+$ cells in cord blood

	Increase $CD34^+$ cells	Decrease $CD34^+$ cells
Gestational age	Younger	Older
Birth weight	Heavier	Lighter
Mother's age	Inconsistent results	Inconsistent results
Baby's sex	NS	NS
Delivery methods	NS	NS
Collection volume	NS	NS
Race	Caucasian	African-American
Maternal iron status	Normal serum ferritin	Increased serum ferritin
Processing time	10 h or shorter	Longer than 10 h

NS not significant

In contrast, the proportions of endothelial colony-forming cells remained constant until term birth [23].

There is an interesting association between circulating hematopoietic stem cells in preterm cord blood and prematurity complications (e.g., intraventricular hemorrhage, respiratory distress syndrome, infections, and anemia). The higher number of circulating $CD34^+$ cells in neonate has been found to be linked to the lower risk of prematurity-related complications [24]. Although causal relationships have not been established, the circulating hematopoietic stem cells may have protective role for the prematurity complications. Relevant to this hypothesis, the number of circulating $CD34^+$cells was significantly higher in survivor of neonatal respiratory distress syndrome than in non-survivor [25].

8.5 Conclusion

Cord blood is a rich source of stem cells/progenitors for regenerative medicine. The field of cord blood stem cell research has undergone tremendous growth during the past decade. CD34 surface antigen has still been a reliable stemness marker for decades, but newer functional-based "stemness" markers (e.g., ALDH) have emerged. Combinatory use of these markers would be more appropriate for variety of regenerative applications in the near future.

References

1. Keeney M, Chin-Yee I, Weir K, Popma J, Nayar R, Sutherland DR. Single platform flow cytometric absolute CD34+ cell counts based on the ISHAGE guidelines. International Society of Hematotherapy and Graft Engineering. Cytometry. 1998;34:61–70.
2. Wagner JE, Barker JN, DeFor TE, Scott Baker K, Blazar BR, Eide C, et al. Transplantation of unrelated donor umbilical cord blood in 102 patients with malignant and nonmalignant

diseases: influence of CD34 cell dose and HLA disparity on treatment-related mortality and survival. Blood. 2002;100:1611–8.
3. Tavian M, Coulombel L, Luton D, Clemente HS, Dieterlen-Lièvre F, Péault B. Aorta-associated CD34+ hematopoietic cells in the early human embryo. Blood. 1996;87:67–72.
4. Medvinsky A, Rybtsov S, Taoudi S. Embryonic origin of the adult hematopoietic system: advances and questions. Development. 2011;138:1017–31.
5. Tavian M, Hallais MF, Péault B. Emergence of intraembryonic hematopoietic precursors in the pre-liver human embryo. Development. 1999;126:793–803.
6. Slayton WB, Juul SE, Calhoun DA, Li Y, Braylan RC, Christensen RD. Hematopoiesis in the liver and marrow of human fetuses at 5 to 16 weeks postconception: quantitative assessment of macrophage and neutrophil populations. Pediatr Res. 1998;43:774–82.
7. Furness SG, McNagny K. Beyond mere markers: functions for CD34 family of sialomucins in hematopoiesis. Immunol Res. 2006;34:13–32.
8. Cheng J, Baumhueter S, Cacalano G, Carver-Moore K, Thibodeaux H, Thomas R, et al. Hematopoietic defects in mice lacking the sialomucin CD34. Blood. 1996;87:479–90.
9. Suzuki A, Andrew DP, Gonzalo JA, Fukumoto M, Spellberg J, Hashiyama M, et al. CD34-deficient mice have reduced eosinophil accumulation after allergen exposure and show a novel crossreactive 90-kD protein. Blood. 1996;87:3550–62.
10. Bhatia M, Wang JC, Kapp U, Bonnet D, Dick JE. Purification of primitive human hematopoietic cells capable of repopulating immune-deficient mice. Proc Natl Acad Sci U S A. 1997;94:5320–5.
11. Hemmati HD, Nakano I, Lazareff JA, Masterman-Smith M, Geschwind DH, Bronner-Fraser M, et al. Cancerous stem cells can arise from pediatric brain tumors. Proc Natl Acad Sci U S A. 2003;100:15178–83.
12. Takahashi M, Matsuoka Y, Sumide K, Nakatsuka R, Fujioka T, Kohno H, et al. CD133 is a positive marker for a distinct class of primitive human cord blood-derived CD34-negative hematopoietic stem cells. Leukemia. 2013;28:1308–15.
13. Salven P, Mustjoki S, Alitalo R, Alitalo K, Rafii S. VEGFR-3 and CD133 identify a population of CD34+ lymphatic/vascular endothelial precursor cells. Blood. 2003;101:168–72.
14. Finney MR, Fanning LR, Joseph ME, Goldberg JL, Greco NJ, Bhakta S, et al. Umbilical cord blood-selected CD133(+) cells exhibit vasculogenic functionality in vitro and in vivo. Cytotherapy. 2010;12:67–78.
15. Balber AE. Concise review: aldehyde dehydrogenase bright stem and progenitor cell populations from normal tissues: characteristics, activities, and emerging uses in regenerative medicine. Stem Cells. 2011;29:570–5.
16. Ma I, Allan AL. The role of human aldehyde dehydrogenase in normal and cancer stem cells. Stem Cell Rev. 2011;7:292–306.
17. Christ O, Lucke K, Imren S, Leung K, Hamilton M, Eaves A, et al. Improved purification of hematopoietic stem cells based on their elevated aldehyde dehydrogenase activity. Haematologica. 2007;92:1165–72.
18. Nakagawa R, Watanabe T, Kawano Y, Kanai S, Suzuya H, Kaneko M, et al. Analysis of maternal and neonatal factors that influence the nucleated and CD34+ cell yield for cord blood banking. Transfusion. 2004;44:262–7.
19. Pope B, Hokin B, Grant R. Effect of maternal iron status on the number of CD34+ stem cells harvested from umbilical cord blood. Transfusion. 2014;54:1876–80.
20. Omori A, Manabe M, Kudo K, Tanaka K, Takahashi K, Kashiwakura I. Influence of obstetric factors on the yield of mononuclear cells, CD34+ cell count and volume of placental/umbilical cord blood. J Obstet Gynaecol Res. 2010;36:52–7.
21. Page KM, Mendizabal A, Betz-Stablein B, Wease S, Shoulars K, Gentry T, et al. Optimizing donor selection for public cord blood banking: influence of maternal, infant, and collection characteristics on cord blood unit quality. Transfusion. 2014;54:340–52.
22. Wisgrill L, Schüller S, Bammer M, Berger A, Pollak A, Radke TF, et al. Hematopoietic stem cells in neonates: any differences between very preterm and term neonates? PLoS One. 2014;9:e106717.

23. Podestà M, Bruschettini M, Cossu C, Sabatini F, Dagnino M, Romantsik O, et al. Preterm cord blood contains a higher proportion of immature hematopoietic progenitors compared to term samples. PLoS One. 2015;10:e0138680.
24. Kotowski MJ, Safranow K, Kawa MPMP, Lewandowska J, Kłos P, Dziedziejko V, et al. Circulating hematopoietic stem cell count is a valuable predictor of prematurity complications in preterm newborns. BMC Pediatr. 2012;12:148.
25. Qi Y, Qian L, Sun B, Chen C, Cao Y. Circulating CD34(+) cells are elevated in neonates with respiratory distress syndrome. Inflamm Res. 2010;59:889–95.

Chapter 9
The History of Hypothermia Therapy for Perinatal Ischemic Brain Injury

Makoto Nabetani and Keisuke Kobata

Abstract Firstly, I mention on pathology of ischemic brain injury, including experimental history of hypothermia. Next, I explain about how clinical trial study starts and proceed to Consensus 2010 in which hypothermia therapy should be recommended for newborns with moderate to severe hypoxic-ischemic encephalopathy (HIE). Next I talk about how hypothermia therapy spreads and could be standardized on the guideline and nationwide online registry system in Japan since Consensus 2010. I explain about some research works about efficacy and criteria of hypothermia therapy. I also introduce unique research about how to control core temperature during transportation in Japan. Finally, I talk about the possibility to start new neuroprotective therapy for newborns with perinatal ischemic brain injury.

Keywords Hypothermia · Hypoxic-ischemic-encephalopathy · HIE Cerebral palsy

9.1 Introduction

Neonatal ischemic brain injury subsequently caused permanent motor deficit "cerebral palsy," and cerebral palsy could be often accompanied with severe other complications such as hearing loss, visual disturbance, epilepsy, hydrocephalus, intellectual disability, behavioral problems, and so on. Neonatal ischemic brain injury includes periventricular leukomalacia (PVL), cerebral infarction, hypoxic-ischemic encephalopathy (HIE), and so on. Especially, HIE is a very serious condition which can occur in around 0.5–2/1000 live births and can result in death and disability. Until the advent of cooling for HIE, there was no therapy other than supportive NICU care. In recent years, however, therapeutic brain hypothermia has become established as the first effective therapy for neonates with HIE [1, 2].

M. Nabetani, M.D., Ph.D. (✉) • K. Kobata, M.D.
Department of Pediatrics, Yodogawa Christian Hospital, 1-7-50, Kunijima, Higashi-yodogawaku, Osaka 533-0024, Japan
e-mail: a103111@ych.or.jp

© Springer Nature Singapore Pte Ltd. 2018

H. Shintaku et al. (eds.), *Cell Therapy for Perinatal Brain Injury*,
https://doi.org/10.1007/978-981-10-1412-3_9

9.2 Pathology of Ischemic Brain Injury

In 1969, Olney discovered excitotoxicity, showing that at least some of the neural cell death caused by hypoxia-ischemia was mediated by excess production of the excitatory neurotransmitter glutamate and that it could be blocked pharmacologically to provide good protection against hypoxic damage [3, 4]. In 1989, Brian Meldrum et al. shifted the paradigm, allowing researchers to consider hypoxic-ischemic damage as a treatable disease [5]. This is described precisely in another chapter.

9.2.1 Experimental History of Hypothermia

In 1989 Ginsberg et al. showed that a short period of hypothermia after hypoxia-ischemia in adult rats reduced excitotoxin generation and produced significant protection in the hippocampus [6, 7].

In 1994, Edwards and Wyatt set about using sophisticated MRS approach to replicate secondary energy failure in piglets and rat pups [8, 9]. And in 1996, Thoresen and Srimanne reported protective effect of hypothermia against brain injury in the neonatal rats [10, 11].

In 1997, we reported that irreversible neuronal cell damage is induced by elevation of intracellular Ca ion concentration that has occurred in sequence after excess production of the excitatory neurotransmitter glutamate in immature and mature rats during ischemia and glucose deprivation. And we also reported that hypothermia therapy was effective on hypoxic or ischemic brain damage of rats to suppress energy loss and elevation of intracellular Ca ion concentration [12, 13].

9.3 History of Clinical Trial

Clinically, In 1997 Marion reported that moderate hypothermia could be effective on adults with traumatic head injury [14]. In 1998 Gunn et al. reported that brain cooling would be safe and could be effective on neonatal HIE [15]. In 2000 Azzopardi and Thoresen reported that therapeutic hypothermia including whole-body cooling also could be safe and effective on infants with HIE [16, 17].

9.3.1 Clinical Situation in Japan

Since then, many facilities started trying undergoing brain cooling for newborns with HIE in Japan. However, hypothermia therapy had been applied to neonatal HIE with originally developed protocols in Japan until 2010. In 2010,

International Liaison Committee on Resuscitation (ILCOR) and International Consensus Conference on Cardiopulmonary Resuscitation and Emergency Cardiovascular Care Science With Treatment Recommendations (CoSTR) documented the new guideline that newborns with moderate to severe HIE should be considered for therapeutic hypothermia (TH) [18]. In this guideline, TH treatment should be consistent with the protocols used in the randomized clinical trials, but the number of centers capable of providing standard cooling was limited in Japan.

9.3.2 Methods

So in July 2010, our taskforce was formed to undergo questionnaire study to clinical leads of registered level-II/III neonatal intensive care units regarding the practice of neonatal encephalopathy in order to elucidate the gap between the standard cooling methods and current practice in Japan [19].

9.3.3 Results

56.2% of 203 units were incapable of offering TH because of the reasons such as the shortage of human/medical resources (85.1%) and limited number of cases (21.1%). Eighty-nine centers provided TH using either selective head cooling (88.8%) or whole-body cooling (11.2%). Various target temperatures and cooling durations were used; 20.2% of the units cooled infants without using purpose-built equipments, whereas 14.6% did not continuously monitor the body temperature. Only 43.8% of the units provided TH. Even in centers where TH was offered, adherence to the standard protocols was extremely poor at that time.

9.3.4 Conclusion

To secure the safety and efficacy, further promotion of the standard cooling protocols is required in 2010.

9.4 Guideline of TH in Japan

In 2011 JSPNM & MHLW Japan Working Group also documented practice guidelines of TH for newborns with HIE [20].

9.4.1 Nationwide Online Case Registry

Based on findings from the primary survey, aggressive action plans were introduced that focused on the formulation of clinical recommendations, facilitation of educational events, and opening of nationwide online case registry. Findings from the follow-up survey (January 2013) were compared with results from the primary survey. Four workshops and three consensus meetings were held to formulate clinical recommendations, which were followed by the publication of practical textbooks, large-scale education seminars, and implementation of a case registry. A follow-up survey covering 253 units (response rate: 89.1%) showed that cooling centers increased from 89 to 135. Twelve prefectures had no cooling centers in 2010, whereas all 47 prefectures had at least 1 in 2013. In cooling centers, adherence to the standard cooling protocols and the use of servo-controlled cooling devices improved from 20.7% to 94.7% and from 79.8% to 98.5%, respectively.

9.4.2 Conclusion

A rapid improvement in the national provision of evidence-based cooling was achieved. International consensus guidelines coupled with domestic interventions might be effective in changing empirical approaches to evidence-based practice [19, 21].

9.5 Efficacy of TH in Japan

9.5.1 Introduction

Unfortunately, in Japan, we could not get any articles that showed the efficacy of TH precisely until consensus 2010. In 2013, we presented first retrospective comparative study in Japan to investigate factors affecting the developmental prognosis of infants with severe neonatal asphyxia who required TH [22].

9.5.2 Methods

We retrospectively reviewed clinical findings of 54 newborns admitted to the Neonatal Intensive Care Unit (NICU) of two hospitals in Japan during September 2004 to May 2010. Total 54 infants with Sarnat classification moderate to severe HIE underwent selective head cooling.

They were divided into two groups according to cognitive findings at 18 months corrected age, using development test. Clinical variables such as birth weight, Apgar scores at 1 and 5 min, body temperature at admission, and time between birth and cooling and pH and base excess (BE) in infant blood on delivery were compared between subjects with full-scale developmental quotients >=70 (Group A, $n = 36$) and <70 (Group B, $n = 18$). The blood samples on delivery were either venous or arterial blood and measured before TH.

9.5.3 Results

There were no adverse effects during TH, and no infant died throughout the study period. Total sex ratio was 1.16, and mean gestational age was 38.8 weeks. The neurodevelopmental outcome of this study participants was assessed with developmental test at corrected 18 months of age by trained assessors, and they were classified by their DQ into DQ > =70 and DQ < 70 groups. Infants of DQ > =70 (Group A) were 36 and DQ < 70 (Group B) were 18, respectively, with developmental test at corrected 18 months of age. Mean birth weights of Groups A and B were 2958 and 2656 g. The body temperatures at admission were 36.4 and 35.9 °C. The pH were 7.04 and 7.05, and BE were −14.7 and −16.6 mmol/L, respectively. There were no significant differences in two groups about these factors. Apgar scores (1 min/5 min) were 3.5/5.0 and 1.7/3.2, and the times between birth and cooling were 218 and 290 min, respectively, and about these factors, there were significant differences in two groups. With logistic regression analysis, only time between birth and cooling significantly related to poor neurologic outcome ($p = 0.04$, odds ratio [OR], 1.235; 95% confidence interval [CI], 1.001–1.524) (Table 9.1).

Table 9.1 Characteristics and outcomes for neonates treated with hypothermia

	DQ > =70 (*N* = 36)	DQ < 70 (*N* = 18)	*p* value	Adjusted OR (95% CI)	Adjusted *p* value
Birth weight, mean ± SD (g)	2958 ± 591	2656 ± 434	0.60	–	–
Apgar score					
1 min	3.5	1.7	0.02	–	–
5 min	5.0	3.2	0.03	0.783 (0.610–1.007)	0.06
Temperature at admission, mean ± SD (°C)	36.4 ± 1.2	35.9 ± 1.9	0.18	–	–
Time between birth and cooling, mean ± SD (min)	218 ± 101	290 ± 110	0.02	1.235 (1.001–1.524)	0.04[a]
pH in infant blood on delivery, mean ± SD	7.04 ± 0.17	7.05 ± 0.20	0.86	–	–
BE in infant blood on delivery, mean ± SD (mmol/L)	−14.7 ± 6.7	−16.6 ± 7.1	0.34	–	–

Statistical analysis
Student's *t*-test is used to compare each factor, and logistic regression analysis was used to investigate confounding between the various factors investigated. In the logistic regression analysis, two groups classified by DQ were specified as dependent variables, and Apgar score (5 min) and time between birth and cooling were specified as independent variables

9.5.4 *Conclusion*

The results demonstrated that the shorter the interval between birth and starting TH, the better the prognosis. The time between birth and cooling would be one of an essential factor in improving outcome for newborns with hypoxic-ischemic encephalopathy. The 1- and 5-min Apgar scores both significantly affected prognosis, but no significance was found on logistic analysis. We need further investigation regarding the effects of the 10-minute Apgar scores, which are indicated to strongly influence neurological prognosis [23]. And further investigation will be conducted on a larger study population connecting with nationwide online case registry and will include longer-term prognoses.

9.6 Regional Network and Establishment of Transportation System

9.6.1 *Introduction*

TH has been shown to improve survival and neurodevelopmental outcome following perinatal asphyxia [2, 24]. To obtain the maximum benefit, TH should be initiated as soon as possible and within 6 h after birth. Particularly, outborn infants might not be able to transport to cooling center and initiate TH within 6 h. Furthermore, it is thought that elevated core temperature after asphyxial insults is associated with worse outcomes among HIE infants [25]. Therefore, it is truly essential to develop effective and safe methods of cooling during transport, because over half of babies were born in private clinics in Japan. Passive cooling could be a simple technique to prevent brain damage from HIE during transport [26–28]. However, we have not got useful device to monitor core temperature during transport. Therefore, we have evaluated how to control core and skin temperature of infants with/without asphyxia during transport from clinics to hospitals in Japan in this study [29].

9.6.2 *Objective*

To evaluate the efficacy and safety of continuous monitoring of rectal temperatures during transport of infants with/without asphyxia in order to control body temperature properly and to induce passive cooling for infants with mild to severe HIE safely.

9.6.3 Methods

Skin and rectal temperatures during transport were prospectively collected from transported newborns between August 2012 and August 2014 at three regional cooling centers. In the case of infants without asphyxia, the transport team controlled the temperature of the transport incubator 33 ± 2 °C to maintain a target rectal temperature at as close to 36.0–36.5 °C as possible. While in the case of infants with asphyxia, the transport team controlled the temperature of the transport incubator between 31 and 32 °C to maintain a target rectal temperature at as close to 35.0 °C as possible.

9.6.4 Results

In the 2-year study period, the skin and rectal temperatures of 52 newborns without asphyxia were monitored continuously. The median gestational age and birth weight of them were 38.1 (36.0–41.3) weeks and 2905 (1904–4408) g. The rectal temperature is correlated significantly with skin temperature ($p < 0.001$) (Fig. 9.1). In two cases, only rectal temperatures but skin temperatures showed decrease (≥0.4 °C) in winter season (Fig. 9.2).

Twelve infants with asphyxia were passively cooled during transport. Ten of twelve cases were analyzed. The median gestational age and birth weight of them were 39.6 (34.0–41.0) weeks and 2584 (2032–2838) g. Six cases of ten showed

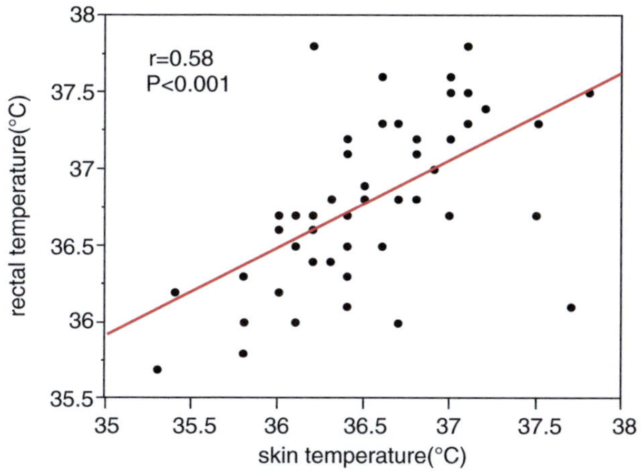

Fig. 9.1 Correlation between rectal and skin temperature of 52 infants without asphyxia

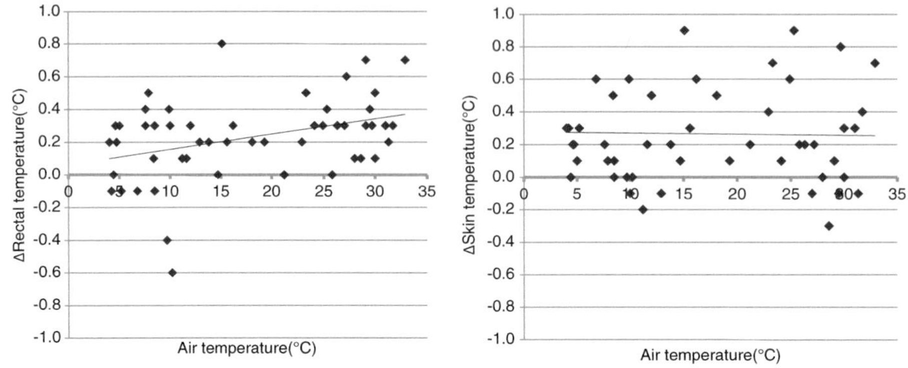

Fig. 9.2 The relationship between rectal or skin temperature change and air temperature

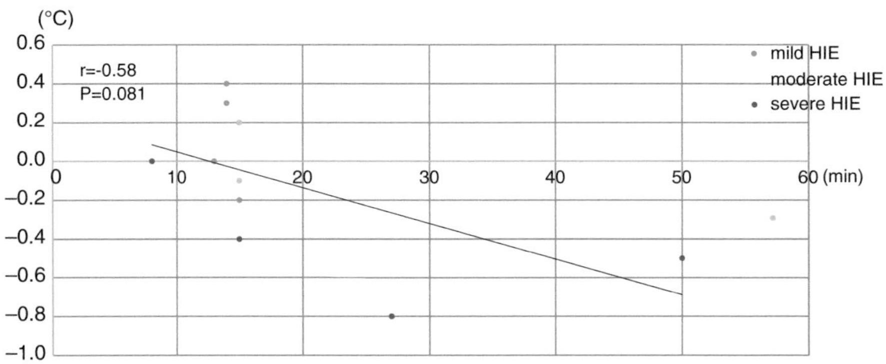

Fig. 9.3 The association between rectal temperature change and journey time

moderate or severe HIE and four cases of ten showed mild HIE. The median rectal temperature at arrival was 35.3 (32.9–36.4) °C (NS). Four of six moderate or severe HIE infants had a rectal temperature at arrival between 34.5 and 35.5 °C and one >35.5 °C. One of four mild HIE infants had a rectal temperature at arrival between 34.5 and 35.5 °C and three >35.5 °C. Only one preterm infant with severe HIE was overcooled.

9.6.5 Conclusion

Passive cooling by controlling the transport incubator temperature for infants with HIE was relatively safe and could prevent to be elevated body temperature. However, there may be a risk of unintended excessive cooling, especially in severe HIE infants and preterm infants during longer transfer (Fig. 9.3). We suggest that continuous monitoring of the rectal temperature to control body temperature during transport especially in the cases which need passive cooling is mandatory.

9.7 Inclusion and Exclusion Criteria

9.7.1 Introduction

It is unknown whether other neonatal patient groups could benefit from TH. So, Thoresen has offered cooling to infants fulfilling the standard cooling criteria but also to those who did not since 2006 [30]. Observational study with prospective data collection over a 6-year period in a regional cooling center. Complications and outcome were compared between infants who were cooled not fulfilling the standard inclusion criteria and exclusion criteria as set out in CoolCap/Toby protocols (n = 36) and infants who fulfilled the standard entity criteria (n = 129). 21.8% of cooled infants did not fulfill standard entity criteria. The induced infants cooled >6 postnatal hours, late preterm infants, and infants with postnatal collapse, major cranial hemorrhage, congenital cardiac disease, and surgical conditions. Complication rates and long-term outcome did not differ significantly between the groups, apart from in infants with a major cranial hemorrhage who had higher rates of coagulopathy and the worst outcome (80% death/disability). They concluded that cooling can be considered for infants with neonatal encephalopathy following postnatal collapse or preterm birth, those with underlying surgical or cardiac conditions, and infants starting cooling >6 postnatal hours.

9.7.2 Objective

On the other hand, many institutions give up to start TH therapy in the HIE case with PPHN. They have regarded PPHN as one of exclusion criteria of TH therapy since there have been a few reports that PPHN cases with moderate to severe HIE cases could undergo TH therapy safely. However, we have experienced six PPHN cases with moderate to severe HIE who could undergo TH therapy safely combined with NO therapy [31].

We have reported experiences of therapeutic hypothermia therapy on six cases with PPHN and moderate to severe HIE using NO therapy. The aim of this study is to clarify whether PPHN is exclusion criteria of TH therapy or not. We studied about seven cases with neonatal moderate to severe HIE using TH therapy combined with NO therapy.

9.7.3 Methods

We experienced six PPHN cases which could undergo TH therapy combined with NO therapy and one PPHN case which could undergo and stop TH during 2002–2014 in Yodogawa Christian Hospital. We experienced no complication in these six cases. No case showed methemoglobinemia or cerebral hemorrhage during TH and NO therapy in these seven cases. We have compared these factors such as gestational age, Apgar score (1 min), Apgar score (10 min), another combined therapy, MRI findings around 1 year of age, GMFCS, and developmental quotient around 1.5 years of age in TH group (38 cases) with those in TH + NO group (6 cases).

9.7.4 Results

There are no significant differences of perinatal factors, MRI findings, GMFCS, and developmental quotient between TH + NO group and TH group (Figs. 9.4, 9.5, and 9.6). All of six cases have used vasoactive agonists; three of six cases have used vasodilators. All of six cases had succeeded to recover from PPHN condition. These results showed TH could be performed safely for HIE cases with PPHN combined with NO therapy maintaining the stable condition of respiration and circulation. We need to investigate more PPHN cases with NO therapy to clarify criteria which cases could be performed TH therapy safely.

9.7.5 Conclusion

We could show the possibility to undertake TH therapy safely for newborns with HIE and PPHN who need NO therapy, if we could maintain intensive respiratory and cardiac support carefully. Even in the most severe brain condition, TH therapy did not deteriorate circulatory and respiratory condition. We need multicentered investigations to clarify more precise entry criteria and exclusion criteria of TH therapy for newborns with moderate to severe HIE.

Now also in Japan, new clinical study on inclusion and exclusion criteria of TH is ongoing in order to protect more infants from perinatal brain injury. Furthermore, clinical studies of new neuroprotective therapies including xenon gas therapy, autologous cord blood therapy, and mesenchymal stem cell therapy have started all over the world. I feel that hypothermia therapy has opened new gate to progress neuroprotective therapy for infants with perinatal brain injury.

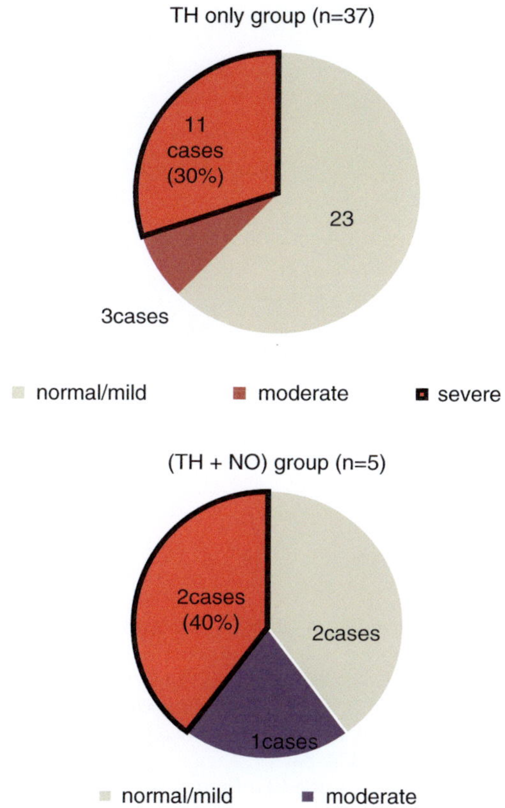

Fig. 9.4 Brain MRI findings at 1 year old

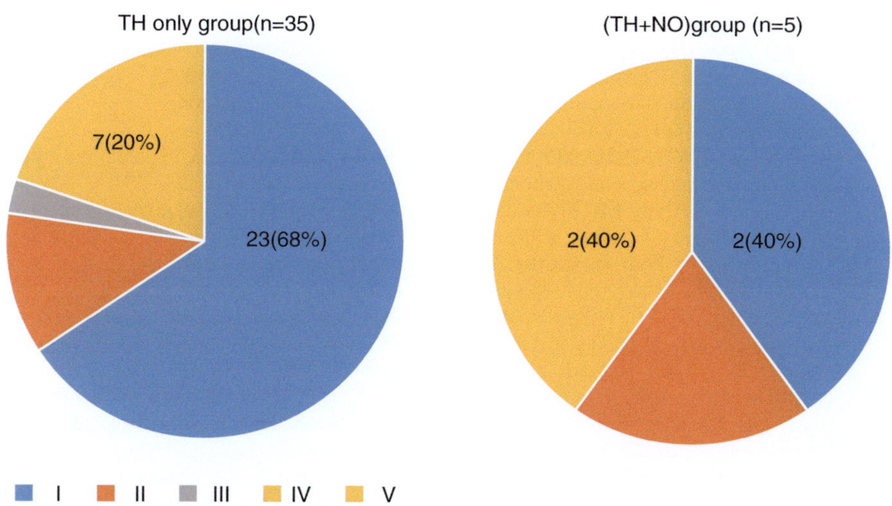

Fig. 9.5 GMFCS at 1.5 years old

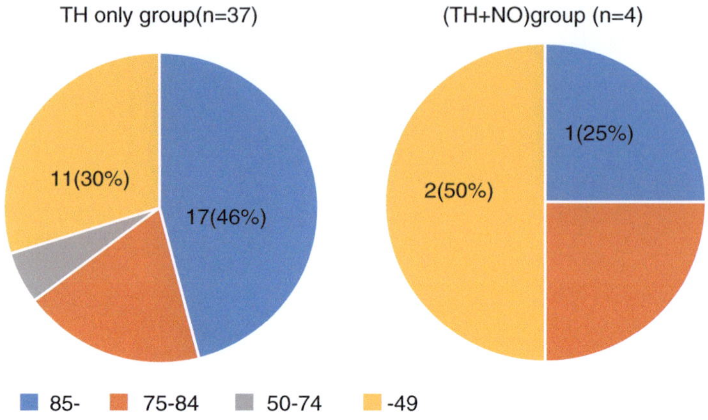

Fig. 9.6 Developmental quotient at 1.5 years old

References

1. Gluckman PD, Wyatt JS, Azzopardi D, Ballard R, Edwards AD, Ferriero DM, et al. Selective head cooling with mild systemic hypothermia to improve neurodevelopmental outcome following neonatal encephalopathy. Lancet. 2005;365:663–70.
2. Shankaran S, Laptook AR, Ehrenkranz RA, Tyson JE, McDonald SA, Donovan EF, et al. Whole-body hypothermia for neonates with hypoxic-ischemic encephalopathy. N Engl J Med. 2005;353:1574–84.
3. Olney JW, Sharpe LG. Brain lesions in an infant rhesus monkey treated with monosodium glutamate. Science. 1969;166:386–8.
4. Olney JW, Ho OL. Brain damage in infant mice following oral intake of glutamate, aspartate or cysteine. Nature. 1970;227:609–11.
5. Simon RP, Swan JH, Griffiths T, Meldrum BS. Blockage of N-methyl-D-aspartate receptors may protect against ischemic damage in the brain. Science. 1984;226:850–2.
6. Enhoming G, Westin B. Experimental studies of the human fetus in prolonged asphyxia. Acta Physiol Scand. 1954;31:359–75.
7. Busto R, Dietrich WD, Globus MY, Ginsberg MD. Postischemic moderate hypothermia inhibits CA1 hippocampal ischemic neuronal injury. Neurosci Lett. 1989;101:299–304.
8. Lorek A, Takei Y, Cady EB, Wyatt JS, Penrice J, Edwards AD, et al. Delayed ("secondary") cerebral energy failure following acute hypoxia-ischemia in the newborn piglets: continuous 48-hour studies by 31P magnetic resonance spectroscopy. Pediatr Res. 1994;36:699–706.
9. Blumberg RM, Cady EB, Wigglesworth JS, JE MK, Edwards AD. Relation between delayed impairment of cerebral energy metabolism and infraction following transient focal hypoxia ischemia in the developing brain. Exp Brain Res. 1996;113:130–7.
10. Thoresen M, Begenholm R, Loberg EM, Apricena F, Kjellmer I. Posthypoxic cooling of neonatal rats provides protection against brain injury. Arch Dis Child Fetal Neonatal Ed. 1996;74:F3–9.
11. Srimanne E, Blumberg RM, Bossano D, Gunning M, Edwards AD, Gluckman PD, et al. The effect of prolonged modifying of cerebral temperature on outcome following hypoxic-ischemic brain injury in the infant rat. Pediatr Res. 1996;39:591–7.
12. Nabetani M, Okada Y, Takata T, Takada S, Nakamura H. Neural activity and intracellular Ca2+ mobilization in the CA1 area of hippocampal slices from immature and mature rats during ischemia and glucose deprivation. Brain Res. 1997;769:158–62.

13. Takata T, Nabetani M, Okada Y. Effects of hypothermia on the neuronal activity, [Ca2+]I accumulation and ATP levels during oxygen and/or glucose deprivation in hippocampal slices of guinea pigs. Neurosci Lett. 1997;227:41–4.
14. Marion DW, Penrod LE, Kelsey SF, Obrist WD, Kochanek PM, Palmer AM, et al. Treatment of traumatic brain injury with moderate hypothermia. N Engl J Med. 1997;336:540–6.
15. Gunn AJ, Gluckman PD, Gunn TR. Selective head cooling in newborn infants following perinatal asphyxia: a safety pilot study. Pediatrics. 1998;102:885–992.
16. Azzopardi D, Robertson NJ, Cowan FM, Rutherford MA, Rampling M, Edwards AD. Pilot study of treatment with whole body hypothermia for neonatal encephalopathy. Pediatrics. 2000;106:684–94.
17. Thoresen M, Whitelaw A. Cardiovascular changes during mild therapeutic hypothermia and rewarming in infants with hypoxic-ischemic-encephalopathy. Pediatrics. 2000;106:92–9.
18. Perlman JM, Wyllie J, Kattwinkel J, Atkins DL, Chameides L, Goldsmith JP, et al. Neonatal resuscitation: 2010 International Consensus on Cardiopulmonary Resuscitation and Emergency Cardiovascular Care Science With Treatment Recommendations. Circulation. 2010;122:S516–38.
19. Iwata O, Nabetani M, Takenouchi T, Iwaibara T, Iwata S, Tamura M. Working group on therapeutic hypothermia for neonatal encephalopathy, Ministry of Health, Labor and Welfare, Japan; Japan Society for Perinatal and Neonatal Medicine. Hypothermia for neonatal encephalopathy: Nationwide Survey of Clinical Practice in Japan as of August 2010. Acta Paediatr. 2012;101(5):e197–202.
20. Takenouchi T, Iwata O, Nabetani M, Tamura M. Therapeutic hypothermia for neonatal encephalopathy: JSPNM & MHLW Japan working group practice guidelines consensus statement from the working group on therapeutic hypothermia for neonatal encephalopathy, Ministry of Health, Labor and Welfare (MHLW), Japan, and Japan Society for Perinatal and Neonatal Medicine (JSPNM). Brain and Development. 2012;34(2):165–70.
21. Tsuda K, Mukai T, Iwata S, Shibasaki J, Tokuhisa T, Ioroi T, et al. Therapeutic hypothermia for neonatal encephalopathy: a report from the first 3 years of the Baby Cooling Registry of Japan. Sci Rep. 2017;7:39508. https://doi.org/10.1038/srep39508.
22. Mukai T, Nabetani M. The factors affecting prognosis for development in newborns with hypoxic ischemic encephalopathy after therapeutic hypothermia. PAS Annual Meeting, 2012, Boston.
23. Laptook AR, Shankaran S, Ambalavanan N, Carlo WA, McDonald SA, Higgins RD, et al. Outcome of term infants using apgar scores at 10 minutes following hypoxic-ischemic encephalopathy. Pediatrics. 2009;124(6):1619–26.
24. Azzopardi DV, Strohm B, Edwards AD, Dyet L, Halliday HL, Juszczak E, et al. Moderate hypothermia to treat perinatal asphyxial encephalopathy. N Engl J Med. 2009;361:1349–58.
25. Laptook AR, Tyson JE, Shankaran S, McDonald SA, Ehrenkranz RA, Fanaroff A, et al. Elevated temperature after hypoxic-ischemic encephalopathy: risk factor for adverse outcomes. Pediatrics. 2008;122:491–9.
26. Anerson ME, Longhofer TA, Phillips W, McRay DE. Passive cooling to initiate hypothermia for transported encephalopathic newborns. J Perinatol. 2007;27:592–3.
27. Hallberg B, Olson L, Bartocci M, Edqvist I, Blennow M. Passive induction of hypothermia during transport of asphyxiated infants: a risk of excessive cooling. Acta Paediatr. 2009;98:942–6.
28. Kendall GS, Kapetanakis A, Ratnavel N, Azzopardi D, Robertson NJ. Passive cooling for initiation of therapeutic hypothermia in neonatal encephalopathy. Arch Dis Child Fetal Neonatal Ed. 2010;95:F408–12.
29. Uemura H, Ioroi T, Nabetani M, Egawa T, Kugo M, Sano H. Takahashi A, Watabe S and Tamura M. Temperature control of infants with/without asphyxia during transport. Neonatal Pediatr Med. 2015;1:1. doi: 10.4172/2572-4983.1000103
30. Smit E, Liu X, Jary S, Cowan F, Thoresen M. Cooling neonates who do not fulfill the standard cooling criteria-short- and long-term outcomes. Acta Pediatr. 2015;104:138–45.
31. Kobata K, Nabetani M, Yutaka N, Hiroyuki, Sanno. Experiences of therapeutic hypothermia therapy on six cases with PPHN and moderate to severe HIE using NO therapy. Int J Neonatal Biol. 2015;4:198.

Chapter 10
Clinical Procedure of Cell Therapy: Cord Blood Collection

Shunsuke Kawahara and Masaaki Hasegawa

Abstract The safety and efficacy of providing umbilical cord blood (UCB) cells to neonates with hypoxic-ischemic encephalopathy (HIE) have recently been reported in the United States (Michael et al. J Pediatr 164:973–979, 2014). We have thus decided to initiate a similar clinical trial in Japan and set obstetric criteria for the indication of cell therapy. Written consent for UCB collection was obtained following successful collection, as the cases included in the study were very limited. Because UCB cells are first administered to neonates 24 h after collection, a more stringent level of aseptic manipulation is required although UCB collection itself is a common procedure in Japan. Therefore, UCB collection was performed ex utero at the proximal end of the umbilical cord because the umbilical vein offers a steady site of puncture at this point, enabling reproducible aseptic UCB collection.

Keywords Cord blood collection · Hypoxic-ischemic encephalopathy
Hematopoietic stem cell · Placental delivery

10.1 Introduction

The safety and efficacy of providing umbilical cord blood (UCB) cells to neonates with hypoxic-ischemic encephalopathy (HIE) have recently been reported in the United States [1], so we have thus decided to initiate a similar clinical trial in Japan.

S. Kawahara, M.D. (✉)
Department of Obstetrics and Gynecology, Kurashiki Central Hospital, Kurashiki-shi, Okayama, Japan

Department of Gynecology and Obstetrics, Graduate School of Medicine, Kyoto University, Kyoto, Japan
e-mail: skawahara@kuhp.kyoto-u.ac.jp

M. Hasegawa, M.D., Ph.D.
Department of Obstetrics and Gynecology, Kurashiki Central Hospital, Kurashiki-shi, Okayama, Japan

© Springer Nature Singapore Pte Ltd. 2018

H. Shintaku et al. (eds.), *Cell Therapy for Perinatal Brain Injury*,
https://doi.org/10.1007/978-981-10-1412-3_10

Cord blood banks consist of public and private cord banks. Public cord banks, which are the source of cells used in hematopoietic stem cell (HSC) transplantation indicated in hematological malignancies, only exist in certain areas [2–6], and UCB collection is performed only in hospitals within an accessible distance. Private cord banks, on the other hand, perform UCB collection and preserve the collected HSCs for potential future use by the neonate or his/her family. UCB collection in the latter case is performed under contract between a private company and a willing individual at the hospital designated by the individual.

The first public cord bank in Japan was established in 1999, and both the number of UCB collection and transplantation are since on the rise [2]. Public cord banks are often situated in urban areas. Because there are no public cord banks in proximity, our hospital is not a UCB collection facility. In initiating the present clinical trial, we thus began by establishing a safe and reproducible protocol for UCB collection.

10.2 Indication

The indication for cell therapy follows that of initiating systemic hypothermia for HIE neonates [7]. Neonates with a congenital anomaly, severe intracranial hemorrhage, birth weight below 1800 g, severe infection, and/or hyperkalemia, neonates born outside of our hospital, and cases in which collected UCB volume was below 40 mL were excluded from the study. UCB collection must be performed on cases satisfying the abovementioned criteria, but such cases are extremely rare. Obstetric criteria to select for such cases thus were set as follows:

1. Cases requiring crash cesarean section under general anesthesia due to non-reassuring fetal status (NRFS).
2. Cases requiring quasi-emergency cesarean section under spinal anesthesia due to NRFS.
3. In cases of vaginal delivery, indication is decided upon maternal and neonatal status after delivery.

10.3 Method of Collection

There are mainly two strategies for UCB collection: collection done while the placenta is in utero or after placental delivery ex utero. We have adopted the ex utero strategy, because it is more technically reproducible, thus rendering the risk of bacterial contamination or clotting lower than in utero [8]. The first administration of collected UCB cells is done 24 h following collection. Infectious disease testing therefore is infeasible within this timeframe, and thus UCB collection must be more carefully performed than for general collection for cord banks. In initiating this clinical trial, we were trained by a skilled doctor from a UCB collection facility and established the following protocol.

Cord blood collection bags, a tube sealer, a pair of roller pliers, and a scale were made readily available in the delivery room (Fig. 10.1) and transported to the operation room by midwives in cases of cesarean section. The above equipment and a clean draped medical cart (Fig. 10.2) were made ready by the time of delivery. The collection bag was placed on the scale, and a portion of the collection tube was fixed onto the cart (Fig. 10.3).

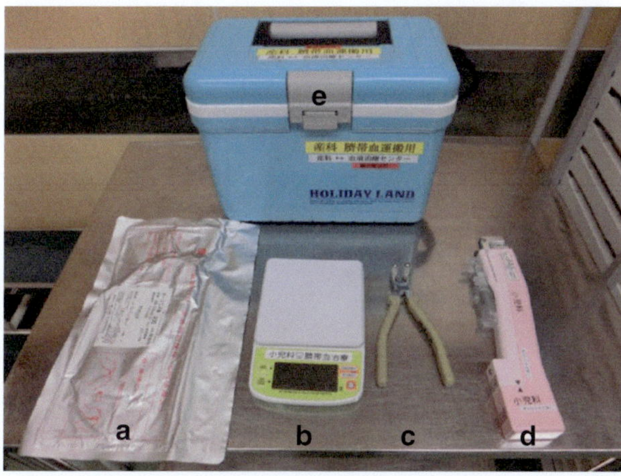

Fig. 10.1 Equipment necessary for umbilical cord collection. Packaged cord blood collection bag (**a**), scale (**b**), a pair of roller pliers (**c**), and a tube sealer (**d**) are stored in a box (**e**) for facile transport and made readily available in the delivery room

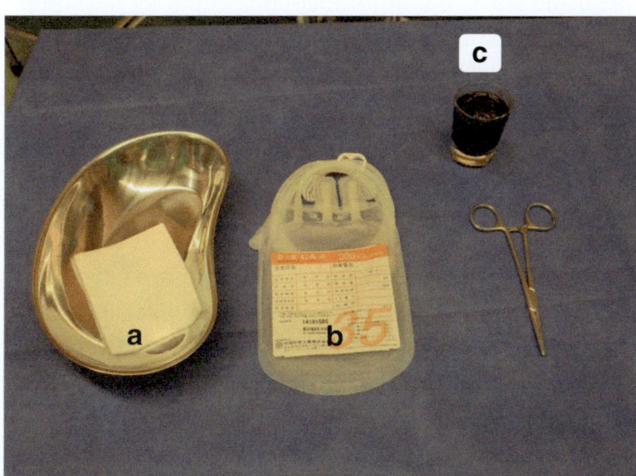

Fig. 10.2 A typical setup, part 1. A piece of gauze drenched in ethanol (**a**), cord blood collection bag taken out of the package (**b**), iodine-povidone cotton swabs (**c**) placed on a clean draped medical cart

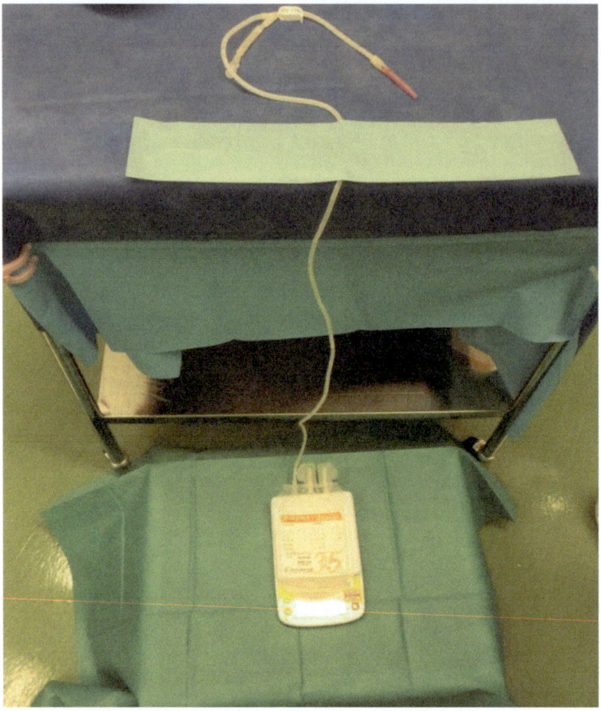

Fig. 10.3 A typical setup, part 2. The collection bag is placed on the scale, and a portion of the collection tube is fixed onto the medical cart

After delivery of the baby, the umbilical cord is cut as proximal to the baby as possible to retain maximal volume of cord blood, and blood gas is obtained from the umbilical artery in utero. The placenta is then detached and transported to the clean draped tray. The umbilical cord is then scrubbed with ethanol and cleaned with a povidone-iodine swab. After waiting for the povidone-iodine to completely dry (to prevent contamination of cord blood by povidone-iodine), the proximal portion of the umbilical vein was punctured with an 18 gauge needle (Fig. 10.4). The site of venipuncture was not manipulated after needle entry. UCB was collected by gravity while occasionally rotating the needle within the umbilical vein. To collect cord blood distal to the site of puncture, the umbilical cord was held above the puncture. Each collection takes 2–4 min [9]. Second punctures were not performed. The proximal portion of the umbilical vein was selected as the site of puncture because the umbilical vein offers a steady site of puncture. Thus, the umbilical vein is less likely to collapse, making reproducible collection possible. The collection bag containing anticoagulants was agitated during the procedure to prevent coagulation. The collection tube was sealed and cut after collection, and the bag was promptly refrigerated at 4 degrees for storage after weighing.

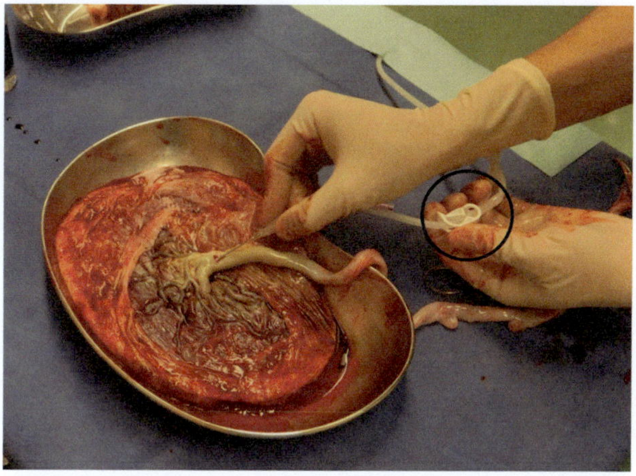

Fig. 10.4 The site of venipuncture. The proximal portion of the umbilical vein was punctured with an 18 gauge needle. After venipuncture, the clamped collection tube (circled) was released. After collection, the needle was removed after re-clamping the collection tube. Second punctures were not performed

10.4 Training

We tested the above protocol before actual clinical implementation on ten cesarean sections and three vaginal deliveries after obtaining consent with documents identical to the ones to be used. In each case, venipuncture was performed by a single doctor, but multiple doctors participated to check the procedure, and each doctor actually performed venipuncture at least once. The average collected volume was 73.8 mL (37–122). All cases were negative of contamination and coagulation (Table 10.1).

10.5 The Issue of Obtaining Consent for UCB Collection

Though the umbilical cord and placenta are often regarded as waste material and discarded, thorough explanation to and written consent of both parents are necessary for UCB collection and transplantation. When to obtain consent is an issue, with consent being obtained before labor, during labor, and after collection in the United States depending on the facility or individual patient details [10].

In Japan, for cord blood donation to public cord banks, consent is generally obtained during prenatal visits. The advantage of obtaining consent before labor is that women are more likely to be relaxed and more able to attend to the issues regarding collection which is necessary for patient-physician rapport. However, the

Table 10.1 Clinical implementation

	Mode of delivery	Weeks of pregnancy	Blood volume (mL)	Birth weight (g)	Placental weight (g)	Coagulation	Contamination
1	CS	38w6d	88	3340	560	None	None
2	CS	38w2d	108	3225	751	None	None
3	CS	38w2d	57	2860	443	None	None
4	CS	38w4d	37	3010	432	None	None
5	CS	39w5d	90	2540	490	None	None
6	CS	38w3d	43	3030	458	None	None
7	CS	38w4d	50	3065	420	None	None
8	CS	38w4d	55	3110	415	None	None
9	CS	39w0d	120	2885	600	None	None
10	CS	37w3d	79	2845	478	None	None
11	VD	37w4d	122	3010	637	None	None
12	VD	38w0d	40	3219	501	None	None
13	VD	41w0d	71	3010	486	None	None

CS cesarean section, *VD* vaginal delivery

inclusion criteria of the present clinical trial are very exclusive and potentially include emergency cases not managed at our hospital, making prior consent difficult. Furthermore, a substantial fraction of the cases included in this clinical trial are likely emergencies, and an unsuccessful collection after prior consent may disappoint willing patients. Weighing the abovementioned possibilities, we have adopted a policy to obtain consent from both patients after successful collection. We have obtained written consent in all cases including training cases and cases in which the patient was found not to meet the inclusion criteria following collection. When a case met the inclusion criteria, a pediatrician has again obtained consent.

10.6 Case Report

The patient was a primipara, naturally conceived and 25 years of age, whose prenatal checkups at another facility were unremarkable. At 38 weeks of gestation, she was admitted to the previous facility due to onset of labor. Because cardiotocogram (CTG) revealed frequent severe late decelerations, a diagnosis of fetal distress was made, and the patient was transferred to our hospital. Pelvic examination at the time of admission revealed vertex position of the fetus, cervical dilatation of 3 cm, and 70 percent effacement. The placenta was fundal, and a 7.6 × 3.9 cm area of high brightness presumably due to hematoma was observed between the placenta and the anterior uterine wall upon transabdominal ultrasound. Baseline fetal heart rate was 170 bpm with reduced variability, and accelerations were absent. Placental abruption was suspected, the patient underwent emergency cesarean section under general anesthesia, and the decision to perform UCB collection was made simultaneously. As previously designated, midwives transported necessary equipment and an incubator to the operation room. The baby was delivered in 4 min. The baby boy weighed 2436 g with an Apgar score of 2 (2 for pulse) at 1 min and 5 (2 for pulse, 1 for muscle tone, 1 for responsiveness, 1 for appearance) at 5 min and an umbilical artery pH of 7.225. The baby was intubated 10 min after birth. Couvelaire sign on the anterior uterine wall, in concordance with suspicion of placental abruption, was noted. UCB collection was performed promptly after placental delivery, and 77 mL of cord blood was successfully retrieved. The baby later fulfilled criteria to initiate systemic hypothermia. Consent of the patient and her family was obtained, and the baby received the first cord blood cell transplantation in Japan.

10.7 Discussion

UCB collection is a generally performed procedure in Japan, but interfacility and interpersonal variability exist in the collected UCB volume, and training is necessary for proper and successful collection.

To increase collected UCB volume, clamping of the placenta immediately following delivery of the baby is advised [11, 12]. UCB exists not only in the placenta but also in the umbilical cord: thus, the umbilical cord should be cut as distal from the placenta as possible [13]. Controversy exists regarding which collection strategy should be adopted in terms of collected UCB volume, with some reports favoring the in utero technique [14–17], while others have reported no significant difference [8, 18].

In the present clinical trial, the collected UCB blood is administered to the baby in a short timeframe after collection. Thus, contamination of collected UCB blood must be prevented at all costs. We have thus adopted the ex utero technique, because it is more technically reproducible. Furthermore, considering that it is difficult to keep the vulva stringently aseptic in vaginal delivery, the ex utero technique which performs aseptic manipulation after placental delivery seems to be the safer choice. A possible caveat of the ex utero strategy is that placental delivery in vaginal delivery at times is delayed, which may increase the risk of coagulation.

Venipuncture is performed at the distal end of the umbilical cord (farthest from the placenta) in the in utero technique and in most ex utero collections [6, 13, 15, 19], but clotting and umbilical cord collapse are a problem. We thus perform venipuncture at the proximal end of the umbilical cord, a practice impossible in utero, because the umbilical vein at the proximal end offers a steady site of puncture; umbilical cord collapse was not observed in all cases collected. The UCB within the umbilical cord can also be retrieved by gravity by holding the umbilical cord above the site of venipuncture.

The drawback of the ex utero technique is that it requires one extra doctor compared to that in utero. For the in utero technique, one and two doctors suffice for UCB collection in cesarean delivery and vaginal delivery, respectively. In contrast, for the ex utero technique, three doctors are necessary for collection in cesarean delivery and two even for vaginal delivery if maternal conditions are unstable.

Indication of UCB collection must carefully be determined to prevent omitting very rare conditions in which UCB collection should be performed such as severe asphyxia, which is an indication for systemic hypothermia. Furthermore, in highly emergency cases such as the one reported above, prior consensus within the medical team proves quintessential to promptly decide upon and execute collection. At our hospital, we have convened interdisciplinary meetings of obstetricians, pediatricians, midwives, surgical nurses, and laboratory technicians to this end.

Meconium-stained amniotic fluid and chorioamnionitis could be an issue in cases of NRFS, because infection cannot be ruled out. Whether such cases should be included is controversial. However, sepsis is rare even in these cases, and some papers have reported increased total nucleated cell and CD34 positive cell content in cases with the presence of meconium-stained amniotic fluid [20, 21]. We thus consider that these cases may be included unless there is strong suspicion of maternal systemic infection.

10.8 Conclusion

UCB collection had not been performed at our hospital prior to the present clinical trial. We have thus established the above protocol for UCB collection in initiating this clinical trial. Many hospitals perform UCB collection in utero and do not require as stringent aseptic manipulation as our protocol. In continuing the present clinical trial, whether traditional protocols adopted at other facilities suffice in regard to safety warrants investigation.

References

1. Cotten CM, Murtha AP, Goldberg RN, Grotegut CA, Smith PB, Goldstein RF, et al. Feasibility of autologous cord blood cells for infants with hypoxic-ischemic encephalopathy. J Pediatr. 2014;164:973–9.
2. Nishihira H, Kato K, Isoyama K, Takahashi TA, Kai S, Kato S, et al. The Japanese cord blood bank network experience with cord blood transplantation from unrelated donors for haematological malignancies: an evaluation of graft-versus-host disease prophylaxis. Br J Haematol. 2003;120:516–22.
3. Barker JN, Wagner JE. Umbilical-cord blood transplantation for the treatment of cancer. Nat Rev Cancer. 2003;3:526–32.
4. Rebulla P. Cord blood banking 2002: 112,010 of 7,914,773 chances. Transfusion. 2002;42:1246–8.
5. Cord blood banks. Med Lett Drugs Ther. 2001;43:84.
6. Moise KJ Jr. Umbilical cord stem cells. Obstet Gynecol. 2005;106:1393–407.
7. Gluckman PD, Wyatt JS, Azzopardi D, Ballard R, Edwards AD, Ferriero DM, et al. Selective head cooling with mild systemic hypothermia after neonatal encephalopathy: multiple randomized trial. Lancet. 2005;365:663–70.

8. Lasky LC, Lane TA, Miller JP, Lindgren B, Patterson HA, Haley NR, et al. In utero or ex utero cord blood collection: which is better? Transfusion. 2002;42:1261–7.
9. Cord blood banking for potential future transplantation: subject review. American Academy of Pediatrics. Work Group on Cord Blood Banking. Pediatrics. 1999;104:116–8.
10. Vawter DE, Rogers-Chrysler G, Clay M, Pittelko L, Therkelsen D, Kim D, et al. A phased consent policy for cord blood donation. Transfusion. 2002;42:1268–74.
11. Ballen KK, Wilson M, Wuu J, Ceredona AM, Hsieh C, Stewart FM, et al. Bigger is better: maternal and neonatal predictors of hematopoietic potential of umbilical cord blood units. Bone Marrow Transplant. 2001;27:7–14.
12. Donaldson C, Armitage WJ, Laundy V, Barron C, Buchanan R, Webster J, et al. Impact of obstetric factors on cord blood donation for transplantation. Br J Haematol. 1999;106:128–32.
13. Jones J, Stevens CE, Rubinstein P, Robertazzi RR, Kerr A, Cabbad MF. Obstetric predictors of placental/umbilical cord blood volume for transplantation. Am J Obstet Gynecol. 2003;188:503–9.
14. Wong A, Yuen PM, Li K, Yu AL, Tsoi WC. Cord blood collection before and after placental delivery: levels of nucleated cells, haematopoietic progenitor cells, leukocyte subpopulations and macroscopic clots. Bone Marrow Transplant. 2001;27:133–8.
15. Solves P, Moraga R, Saucedo E, Perales A, Soler MA, Larrea L, et al. Comparison between two strategies for umbilical cord blood collection. Bone Marrow Transplant. 2003;31:269–73.
16. Solves P, Mirabet V, Larrea L, Moraga R, Planelles D, Saucedo E, et al. Comparison between two cord blood collection strategies. Acta Obstet Gynecol Scand. 2003;82:439–42.
17. Surbek DV, Visca E, Steinmann C, Tichelli A, Schatt S, Hahn S, et al. Umbilical cord blood collection before placental delivery during cesarean delivery increases cord blood volume and nucleated cell number available for transplantation. Am J Obstet Gynecol. 2000;183:218–21.
18. Sparrow RL, Cauchi JA, Ramadi LT, Waugh CM, Kirkland MA. Influence of mode of birth and collection on WBC yields of umbilical cord blood units. Transfusion. 2002;42:210–5.
19. Joanne K, Anne DL, Jeremy S. Untying the Gordian knot: policies, practices, and ethical issues related to banking of umbilical cord blood. J Clin Invest. 2015;115:2592–7.
20. Solves P, Perales A, Mirabet V, Roig R. Stress factors and umbilical cord blood banking. Transfus Med. 2007;17:205.
21. Solves P, Perales A, Fillol M, Bonilla F, Mirabet V, Roig R. Presence of meconium-stained amniotic fluid in cesarean deliveries increases the total nucleated cell content of umbilical cord blood units. Transfusion. 2009;49:388–9.

Chapter 11
Clinical Procedure of Cell Therapy: Separation and Infusion

Shinichi Watabe and Mariko Sawada

Abstract Umbilical cord blood (UCB) cells could be a useful adjunct intervention for infants with HIE. We report our clinical experience of UCB stem cell transplantation in infants with HIE. We selected patients for UCB stem cell transplantation based on following criteria; (1) moderate or severe HIE according to the classification of Sarnat II or III and Thompson score ≥10 points, (2) gestational age ≥36 weeks, (3) body weight at birth >1800 g, (4) born by cesarean section under general anesthesia, and (5) inborn baby. Cases in which collected UCB volume is below 40 mL were excluded from this trial. Brain hypothermia therapy (BHT) was performed simultaneously under supportive mechanical ventilation with sedative agents (fentanyl citrate and midazolam). After collected UCB, CD34-positive cells were separated by SEPAX-2™ (Biosafe SA, Eysins/Nyon, Switzerland) and were transfused to the babies once a day for 12 h to 3 days.

This treatment was successful and safe in all three cases with no adverse effects. A randomized phase II study to provide further safety, feasibility, and efficacy information among a wider number of sites is warranted.

Keywords Hypoxic-ischemic encephalopathy (HIE) · Brain hypothermia therapy (BHT) · Umbilical cord blood (UCB) cells · CD34 positive cells

11.1 Introduction

Hypoxic-ischemic encephalopathy (HIE) is a common cause of long-term neurological disability in children. Brain hypothermia therapy (BHT) is the only effective treatment for HIE, but in most cases, BHT is supportive [1–4]. Hypothermia targets pathophysiology related to secondary energy failure, including excitatory neurotransmitter release, destructive apoptosis, and "continuum" cell death [5, 6].

S. Watabe, M.D., Ph.D. (✉) • M. Sawada, M.D.
Neonatal Intensive Care Unit, Kurashiki Central Hospital, Kurashiki City, Okayama Prefecture, Japan
e-mail: sw7156@kchnet.or.jp

© Springer Nature Singapore Pte Ltd. 2018

H. Shintaku et al. (eds.), *Cell Therapy for Perinatal Brain Injury*,
https://doi.org/10.1007/978-981-10-1412-3_11

Neonatal rodents injected with human umbilical cord blood (UCB) cells after HIE have improved anatomic and neurobehavioral outcomes, most likely due to paracrine and trophic effects during the hours and days after injury, leading to speculation that UCB cells could be a useful adjunct intervention for human infants with HIE [7–12]. The potential of usage of stem cells to reduce brain damage or promote regeneration is a possibility that has been tested in different central nervous system (CNS) disorders. In this chapter, we report our clinical experience of umbilical cord stem cell transplantation in infants with HIE.

11.2 Patients

We selected patients for umbilical cord stem cell transplantation based on the following criteria:

1. Moderate or severe HIE according to classification of Sarnat II or III and Thompson score ≥10 points.
2. Gestational age ≥36 weeks.
3. Body weight at birth >1800 g.
4. Born by cesarean section under general anesthesia.
5. Inborn baby. Neonates with congenital anomalies, severe intracranial hemorrhage, severe infection, and/or hyperkalemia, neonates born outside of our hospital, and cases in which collected UCB volume is below 40 mL were excluded from this trial.

11.3 Materials and Methods

UCB was collected from newborn infants in collection bags containing citrate phosphate dextrose as an anticoagulant. In all cases, informed consent was received from their parents before this procedure. After collected UCB, CD34-positive cells were separated by SEPAX-2™ (Biosafe SA, Eysins/Nyon, Switzerland). SEPAX-2™ is a fully automated, mobile, closed capability system for the efficient and consistent processing of umbilical cord blood. The advantages of SEPAX-2™ are as follows (Fig. 11.1):

- Highly efficient and consistent cell recovery
- Easy handling and safety of processing
- Full traceability and good manufacturing practice (GMP)

The combination of the compact SEPAX-2™ main processing unit, application-specific software protocols, and single-use kits allows for the controlled separation of cellular products in a fully automated and secured environment. The SEPAX-2™ is a PC-based device that requires no operator intervention during the separation

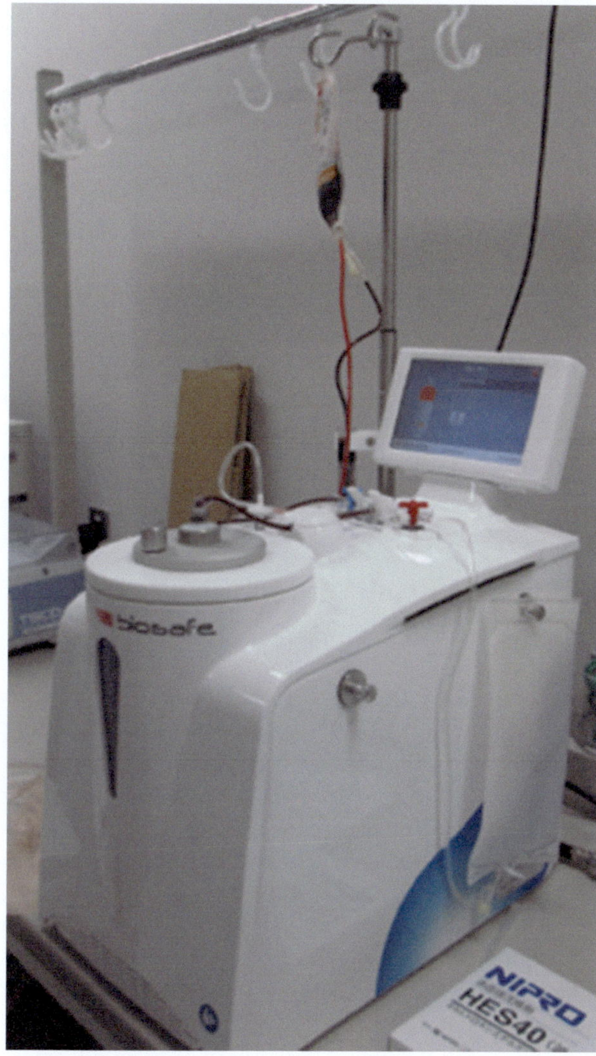

Fig. 11.1 SEPAX-2™ system: SEPAX-2™ is a fully automated, mobile, closed capability system for the efficient and consistent processing of umbilical cord blood

procedure, virtually eliminating operator-influenced processing errors. By this procedure, removal rates of red blood cell (RBC) and plasma are 92% and 79%, respectively, and the recovery percentage of CD34-positive cells is 33%. This low recovery rate of CD34 positive cell might be due to insufficient mixture of package. Hamada reported that recovery percentage of CD34-positive cell was about 90%. A CS-430.1(Biosafe Group SA, Switzerland)separation circuit and UCB-HES separation program are used [13]. After separation of CD34-positive cells, CD34-positive cells are divided into three packages and are transfused to the babies once a day for 12 h to 3 days.

11.3.1 Indications

The indications for cell therapy follow that of initiating systemic hypothermia for HIE neonates. Neonates with a congenital anomaly, severe intracranial hemorrhage, a birth weight below 1800 g, severe infection and/or hyperkalemia, neonates born outside of our hospital, and cases in which the collected UCB volume was below 40 mL were excluded from the study. UCB collection must be performed on cases satisfying the abovementioned criteria, but such cases are extremely rare. Obstetric criteria to select for such cases thus were set as follows:

1. Cases requiring crash cesarean section under general anesthesia due to non-reassuring fetal status (NRFS).
2. Cases requiring quasi-emergency cesarean section under spinal anesthesia due to NRFS.
3. In cases of vaginal delivery, the indications were decided upon maternal and neonatal status after delivery.

11.4 Case Report

11.4.1 Case 1

The patient's mother was a primipara, naturally conceived at 25 years of age. At 38 weeks of gestation, cardiotocogram (CTG) revealed frequent severe late decelerations; thus, a diagnosis of fetal distress was made, and the mother was transferred to our hospital. The placenta was fundal, and a 7.6 × 3.9 cm area of high brightness presumably due to hematoma was observed between the placenta and the anterior uterine wall upon transabdominal ultrasound (Fig. 11.2). Baseline fetal heart rate was 170 bpm with reduced variability, and accelerations were absent. She underwent emergency cesarean section under general anesthesia because placental abruption was suspected. A male neonate was born by cesarean section at 38 weeks of gestation, with a birth weight of 2436 g. After tracheal intubation, the baby was supported with manual ventilation by neonatologists at birth. The Apgar score was 2 points at 1 min, 5 points at 5 min, and 8 points at 15 min. Thirty minutes after birth, the baby was admitted to the neonatal intensive care unit (NICU). The umbilical arterial pH value at birth was 7.255. After delivery, retroplacental hematoma was diagnosed based on histopathological analysis (Fig. 11.3).

The baby was given a diagnosis of Sarnat II HIE. The Thompson HIE score was 12 points (Tables 11.1 and 11.2), which resulted in a diagnosis of moderate HIE. UCB collection was performed promptly after placental delivery, and 77 mL of cord blood was successfully retrieved. Umbilical cord stem cell was centrifuged by SEPAX-2™. The setting of SEPAX-2™ was as follows:

- Centrifuge circuit: CS-430.1
- Centrifugal program: UCB-HES centrifugal program

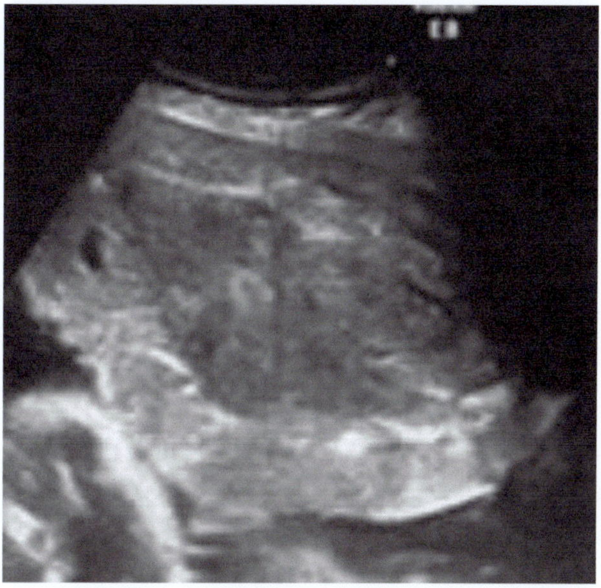

Fig. 11.2 Fetal ultrasonography (case 1): A 7.6 × 3.9 cm area of high brightness presumably due to hematoma was observed between the placenta and the anterior uterine wall on transabdominal ultrasound

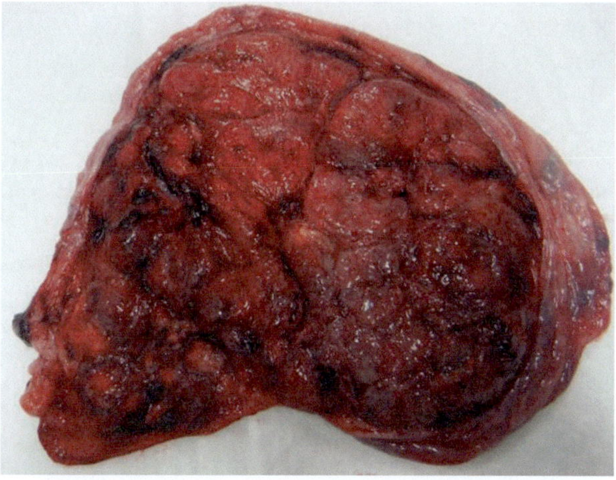

Fig. 11.3 Gross morphology of the placenta (case 1): Weight of placenta was 426 g. Large hematoma was shown on the margin of placenta

A total of 30 mL of CD34-positive cells was recovered after centrifugation which was divided into three packages and transfused to the babies once a day for 1 h during 3 days. No adverse effects occurred during transfusion, and there were no bacteria isolated from any UCB samples.

Table 11.1 Sarnat stage of HIE (case 1): more severe encephalopathy—one or more signs in at least six categories [6]

	Moderate	Severe
Level of consciousness	Lethargic	Stupor or coma
Spontaneous activity	Decreased activity	No activity
Posture	Distal flexion, complete extension	Decerebrate
Tone	Hypotonia (focal or general)	Flaccid
Suck	Week	Absent
Moro	Incomplete	Absent
Pupils	Constricted	Deviated, dilated or non reactive to light
Heart rate	Bradycardia	Variable
Respiration	Periodic breathing	Apnea

This case was given a diagnosis of moderate HIE

Table 11.2 Thompson HIE score (case 1) [14]: total Thompson HIE score was 12 points (moderate HIE)

	1	2	3
Limb tone	Generally hypertonic	Generally hypotonic	Flaccid
Level of consciousness	Hyper alert, hyper-reactive or staring	Lethargic/obtunded	Comatose or stupor
Visible fits	Infrequent <3/day	frequent≧3/day	
Posture	Fisting and/or crying	Strong distil flexion	Decerebrate
Moro	Partial	Absent	
Grasp	Poor	Absent	
Suck	Poor	Absent and/or bites	
Respiratory effort	Hyperventilation	Transient apnea	Apnea
Fontanel	Full	Tense	

11.4.1.1 Evaluation of HIE

Biochemical analysis showed elevations of lactate, creatinine phosphate (CK), and CK-BB (Table 11.3). Brain ultrasound showed a resistance index (RI) in the anterior cerebral artery (ACA) of 0.67 (Fig. 11.4). Amplitude-integrated EEG (a-EEG) showed a moderate suppression-burst pattern.

11.4.1.2 Clinical Course

Brain hypothermia therapy (BHT) was performed simultaneously under supportive mechanical ventilation with sedative agents (fentanyl citrate and midazolam).

The baby was extubated on his 4th day of birth, and oral feeding was started on the 5th day. On the 7th day, oxygen supplementation was stopped, and 30 days after birth, there were no significant findings on brain MRI (Fig. 11.5). But, neuron-specific

Table 11.3 Laboratory data (case 1)

Blood gas analysis(umbilical cord)		
pH	7.225	
Blood gas analysis(venous blood)		
pH	7.218	
pCO_2	48.6	mmol/L
pO_2	49	mmol/L
BE	−7.8	mmol/L
Lactate	7.7	mmol/L
Biochemical data		
CRP	0.049	
Total protein	8.8	g/dL
Alb	3.2	g/dL
AST	87	IU/L
ALT	12	IU/L
Creatinine kinase	771	IU/L
LDH	643	IU/L
Urinary acid	7.2	mg/dL
BUN	8	mg/dL
Na	140	mg/dL
K	5.4	mg/dL
Cl	101	mg/dL
RBC	478×10^4	/μ L
Hct	52.6	%
Hb	17.7	g/dL
WBC	16,800	/μ L
Platelet	19.4×10^4	/μ L
APTT	75.5	s
PT	22	s
PT activity	43	%
PT-INR	1.9	
Peak value of clinical course		
CK	2779	IU/L
CK-BB	71.5	IU/L
Lactate	49.3	mg/dL

enolase (NSE) of cerebrospinal fluid was slightly elevated compared to the standard range (Table 11.3) (Fig. 11.6).

11.4.1.3 Follow-Up

The neuromotor development of this baby is as follows:

Neck hold: 4 months old
Crawling: 6 months old
Sitting: 9 months old
Walking: 1 year old

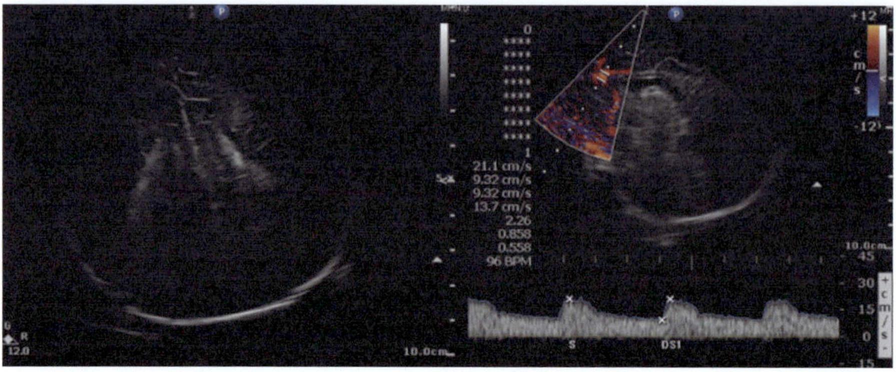

Fig. 11.4 Brain ultrasonography (case 1): There were no findings of brain anomaly and intraventricular hemorrhage (IVH). Resistance index (RI) of anterior cerebral artery (ACA) was 0.67. Amplitude-integrated EEG (a-EEG) showed moderate suppression-burst pattern

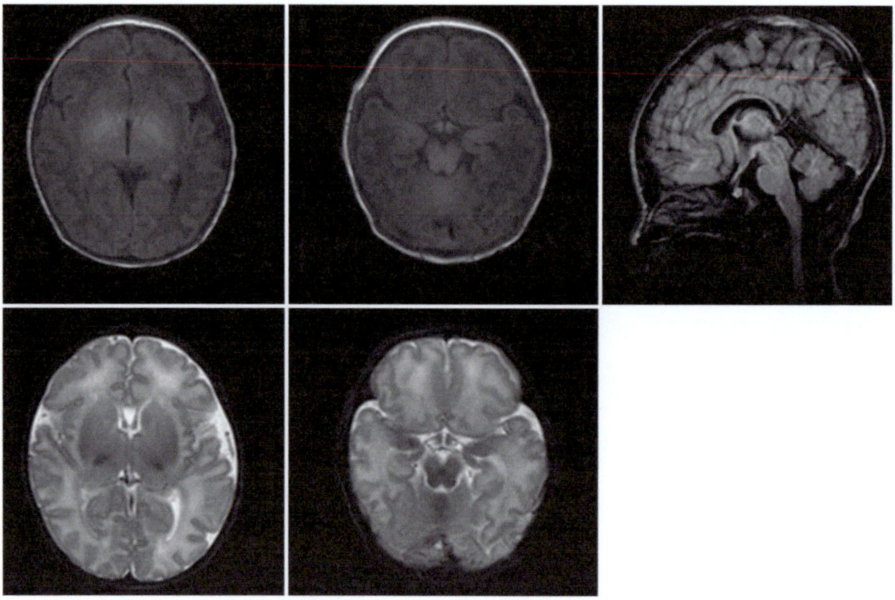

Fig. 11.5 Brain MRI before discharge (case 1). There were no abnormal findings on brain MRI

His total developmental quotient (DQ) by Kyoto Scale of Psychological Development 2001 at 18 months old was 88 points (posture-motor area, 102 points; cognition-adaptation, 85 points; and language society, 89 points). He is suspected of having attention-deficit/hyperactivity disorder (AD/HD).

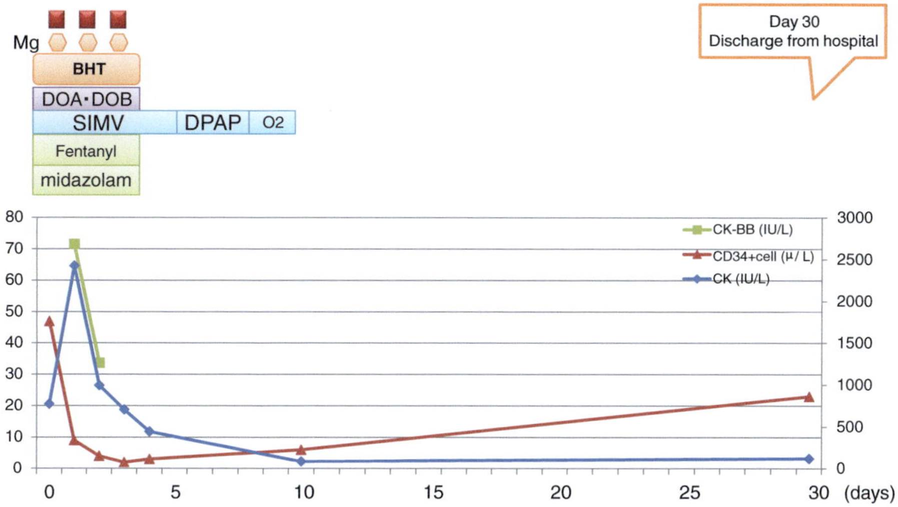

Fig. 11.6 Clinical course of case 1

11.4.2 Case 2

The mother in this case was a unipara, naturally conceived at 28 years of age. At 39 weeks of gestation, CTG revealed frequent severe late decelerations, and a diagnosis of fetal distress was made, resulting in the mother being transferred to our hospital. Despite attempted vaginal delivery, decreasement of the fetal head was difficult, and she underwent emergency cesarean section under general anesthesia. A male neonate was born by cesarean section at 39 weeks of gestation, with a birth weight of 4086 g. The baby was supported with continuous positive airway pressure (CPAP) by neonatologist at birth. After CPAP, the baby started crying and SpO_2 increased to over 80%. After stopping CPAP, SpO_2 decreased to under 90%, and the baby was admitted to NICU. The Apgar score was 5 points at 1 min, 6 points at 5 min, and 9 points at 10 min. Pedaling like seizure occurred 10 min after birth.

The umbilical arterial pH value at birth was 7.230. Thompson HIE score was 12 points. The baby was given a diagnosis of moderate HIE. UCB collection was performed promptly after placental delivery, and 113 mL of cord blood was successfully retrieved. Umbilical cord stem cell was centrifuged, and a total of 18 mL of CD34-positive cells was recovered which was divided into three packages and transfused to the babies once a day for 1 h over 3 days. There were no adverse effects during transfusion. No bacteria were isolated from any UCB sample.

11.4.2.1 Evaluation of HIE

Biochemical analysis showed no elevation of CK-BB, and the resistance index (RI) of the anterior cerebral artery (ACA) was 0.667 by brain ultrasonography. Amplitude-integrated EEG showed a moderate suppression-burst pattern.

11.4.2.2 Clinical Course

BHT was performed simultaneously under supportive mechanical ventilation with sedative agents. On his 30th day of birth, he was discharged from hospital without any apparent complications of UCB transfusion, and there were no remarkable findings on brain MRI. However, neuron-specific enolase (NSE) of cerebrospinal fluid showed a slight elevation than the standard range. At the time of writing, he was 3 months of age, and the neuromotor development of this baby has been within normal limits (eye tracking, 2 months old, and neck hold,4 months old).

11.4.3 Case 3

The mother of case 3 was a primipara, artificially conceived at 31 years of age. At 38 weeks of gestation, she was admitted to our hospital due to a diagnosis of premature rupture of membrane (PROM). Because non-reassuring fetal distress (NRFS) occurred during induction of labor, she underwent emergency cesarean section under general anesthesia. A male neonate was born by cesarean section at 38 weeks of gestation, with a birth weight of 2725 g. After tracheal intubation, the baby was supported with manual ventilation from 3 minute after birth, and the baby was admitted to the NICU. The Apgar scores were 2 points at 1 min, 7 points at 5 min, and 7 points at 10 min, and the umbilical arterial pH value at birth was 7.195. The baby was diagnosed with moderate HIE (Sarnat stage II and Thompson HIE score, 12 points). UCB collection was performed promptly after placental delivery, and 65 mL of cord blood was successfully retrieved. Following centrifuge separation, a total of 18 mL of CD34-positive cells was recovered which was divided into three packages and transfused to the babies for 3 days. No adverse effects are found during transfusion. No bacteria were isolated from the UCB samples.

11.4.3.1 Evaluation of HIE

Biochemical analysis showed no elevation of CK-BB, and resistance index (RI) of the anterior cerebral artery (ACA) was 0.81 by brain ultrasonography. Amplitude-integrated EEG showed a moderate suppression-burst pattern.

11.4.3.2 Clinical Course

BHT was performed simultaneously with CD34 positive cell transfusion. On his 14th day of birth, he was discharged from hospital without any apparent complications of UCB transfusion. There were no remarkable findings on brain MRI. However, neuron-specific enolase (NSE) of cerebrospinal fluid was slightly elevated compared to the standard range. At the time of writing, he was 2 months of age, and the

Table 11.4 Total examination of three cases, which underwent UCB stem cell transplantation

	Case 1	Case 2	Case 3
Lactate (mg/dL)	49.3	20.2	10.3
CK (IU/)	2779	1830	519
CK-BB (IU/L)	71.5	16.5	13.23
Liquor NSE (ng/mL)	62.0	35.0	–
Brain US RI (ACA)	0.67	0.66	0.81
a-EEG	Moderate suppression	Moderate suppression	Moderate suppression
Collected UB volume (mL)	77	113	65
Collected $CD34^+$ volume (mL)	20	18	18
Recovery rate of $CD34^+$	97%	97%	97%
Sarnat stage	II	II	II
Thompson score	12	12	10

neuromotor development of this baby was within the normal range (eye tracking: 2 months old).

A summary of the examination findings of all three cases is shown in Table 11.4.

11.5 Conclusion

We have experienced three cases in which umbilical cord stem cell transplantation was performed in infants with HIE. This treatment was successful and safe in all three cases with no adverse effects. A randomized phase II study to provide further safety, feasibility, and efficacy information among a wider number of sites is warranted.

Acknowledgments The authors thank Yasunori Ueda who is a director of Hematology of Kurashiki Central Hospital, and we also thank comedical staffs of Blood Transfusion and Cell Therapy Department of our hospital.

Conflict of Interest: The authors declare no conflict of interest.

References

1. Gluckman PD, Wyatt JS, Azzopardi D, Ballard D, Edwards AD, Ferriero DM. Selective head cooling with mild systemic hypothermia to improve neurodevelopmental outcome following neonatal encephalopathy. Lancet. 2005;365:663–70.
2. Shankaran S, Laptook AR, Ehrenkranz RA, Tyson JE, McDonald SA, Donovan EF, et al. Whole body hypothermia for neonates with hypoxic-ischemic encephalopathy. N Engl J Med. 2005;35:1574–84.
3. Azzopardi DV, Strohm B, Edwards AD, Dyet L, Halliday HL, Juszczak E, et al. Moderate hypothermia to treat perinatal asphyxial encephalopathy. N Engl J Med. 2009;361:1349–58.

4. Jacobs SE, Morley CJ, Inder TE, Stewart MJ, Smith KR, McNamara PJ, et al. Whole-Body Hypothermia for Term and Near-Term Newborns With Hypoxic-Ischemic Encephalopathy: A Randomized Controlled Trial. Arch Pediatr Adolesc Med. 2011;165:692–700.
5. Gunn AJ, Gunn TR. The pharmacology of neuronal rescue with cerebral hypothermia. Early Hum Dev. 1998;53:19–35.
6. Northington FJ, Zelaya ME, O'Riordan DP, Blomgren K, Flock DL, Hagberg H, et al. Failure to complete apoptosis following neonatal hypoxia-ischemia manifests as "continuum" phenotype of cell death and occurs with multiple manifestations of mitochondrial dysfunction in rodent forebrain. Neuroscience. 2007;149:822–33.
7. Meier C, Middelanis J, Wasielewski B, Neuhoff S, Roth-Haerer A, Gantert M, et al. Spastic paresis after perinatal brain damage in rats is reduced by human cord blood mononuclear cells. Pediatr Res. 2006;59:244–9.
8. Pimentel-Coelho PM, Magalhaes ES, Lopes LM, deAzevedo LC, Santiago MF, Mendez-Otero R. Human cord blood transplantation in a neonatal rat model of hypoxic-ischemic brain damage: functional outcome related to neuroprotection in the striatum. Stem Cells Dev. 2010;19:351–8.
9. Yasuhara T, Hara K, Maki M, Xu L, Yu G, Ali MM, et al. Mannitol facilitates neurotrophic factor up-regulation and behavioural recovery in neonatal hypoxic-ischaemic rats with human umbilical cord blood grafts. J Cell Mol Med. 2010;14:914–21.
10. Geissler M, Dinse HR, Neuhoff S, Kreikemeier K, Meier C. Human umbilical cord blood cells restore brain damage induced changes in rat somatosensory cortex. PLoS One. 2011;6:e20194.
11. Rosenkranz K, Meier C. Umbilical cord blood cell transplantation after brain ischemia—from recovery of function to cellular mechanisms. Ann Anat. 2011;193:371–9.
12. Bennet L, Tan S, Van den Heuij L, Derrick M, Groenendaal F, van Bel F, et al. Cell therapy for neonatal hypoxia-ischemia and cerebral palsy. Ann Neurol. 2012;71:589–600.
13. http://www.haemotec.co.za/category/stem-cell-therapy/biosafe-sepax-automated-cell-processing/
14. Thompson CM, Puterman AS, Linley LL, Hann FM, van der Elst CW, Molteno CD, et al. The value of a scoring system for hypoxic ischaemic encephalopathy in predicting neurodevelopmental outcome. Acta Paediatr. 1997;86(7):757–61.

Chapter 12
Cell Therapy for Adult Infarction

Yasushi Sato, Yukiko Kasahara, and Akihiko Taguchi

Abstract It was believed that neurogenesis does not occur in the adult brain and stroke causes permanent neurological damage without a chance of functional recovery. Recently, accumulating evidences suggest that neurogenesis occurs even in the adult brain and patients may have a chance for functional recovery after stroke. Although most stroke-induced neural stem cells cannot survive in the poststroke brain, we demonstrated that therapeutic angiogenesis after stroke, obtained by intravenous administration of hematopoietic stem cells, supports survival of stroke-induced neural stem cells, followed by functional recovery, in an experimental stroke model. Based on these observations, we conducted a phase 1/2a clinical trial of bone marrow mononuclear cell transplantation in adult patients with cerebral ischemia.

This chapter summarizes the current findings observed in an experimental stroke model regarding cell therapy to enhance function recovery and introduces our clinical trial using autologous bone marrow mononuclear cells for adult patients with cerebral infarction. We also refer to a future strategy of cell therapy that aims to support ideal regenerative process after stroke in the adult brain.

Keywords Cerebral infarction · Neurogenesis · Angiogenesis · Cell therapy Regeneration medicine

12.1 Introduction

Stroke is one of the leading causes of death worldwide and negatively affects the quality of life due to neurological dysfunction. More than 50% of stroke survivors are unable to completely recover, and 20% of patients with stroke require

Y. Sato, Ph.D. • Y. Kasahara, Ph.D. • A. Taguchi, M.D., Ph.D. (✉)
Department of Regenerative Medicine Research, Institute of Biomedical Research and Innovation, Kobe, Japan
e-mail: taguchi@fbri.org

© Springer Nature Singapore Pte Ltd. 2018

H. Shintaku et al. (eds.), *Cell Therapy for Perinatal Brain Injury*,
https://doi.org/10.1007/978-981-10-1412-3_12

assistance with their daily activities. A number of therapies have been attempted to improve stroke outcomes, but no treatment, besides thrombolytic therapy and thrombectomy in the hyperacute phase, has proven to be effective. However, thrombolytic therapy or thrombectomy must be administered within 4.5 or 8 h after stroke onset, respectively [1], and no treatment that improves stroke-induced brain damage exists beyond that period. Thus, novel therapies to regenerate neuronal function and to extend the therapeutic time window after stroke are greatly required [2] (Fig. 12.1).

Recently, cell-based therapies to repair cerebral infarction in adults have been proposed, and their effectiveness has been shown in clinical trials. Since it was believed that the adult mammalian brain does not regenerate, neural stem cell transplantation in patients with stroke was conducted, but it showed only mild or nonsignificant therapeutic effects [3] and some adverse effects [4]. To develop a novel therapeutic strategy for stroke, we investigated the relationship between hematopoietic stem cells and angiogenesis in the brain after stroke and found that angiogenesis is essential for the survival of the stroke-induced neural stem/progenitor cells that contribute to the neurological recovery in postischemic brains. Therefore, we focused on angiogenesis using bone marrow mononuclear cells. This chapter summarizes the findings from basic research on angiogenesis and neurogenesis in post-stroke mammalian brains and introduces phase 1/2a clinical trials that aim to enhance functional recovery in patients following a stroke using therapeutic bone marrow mononuclear cells.

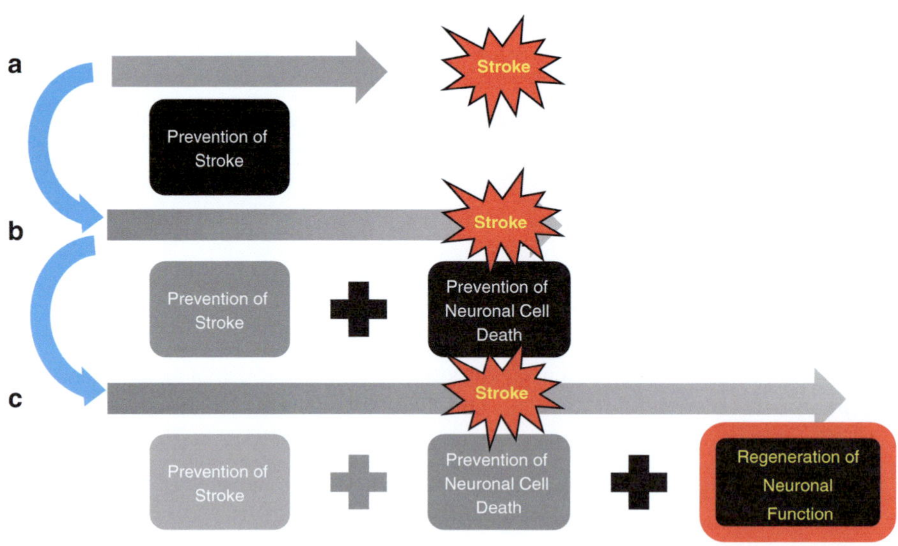

Fig. 12.1 Expansion of the therapeutic time window by cell therapy (Quoted and modified from [2]). As the next strategy after prevention of stroke (**a**) and thrombolysis/thrombectomy (**b**), establishment of novel therapies that extend therapeutic time window is eagerly awaited (**c**)

12.2 Neurogenesis in the Adult Brain

It was believed that the neurons in the adult brain do not regenerate. Recently, it was recognized that neurogenesis continuously occurs in the adult brain. The neurogenesis in the brain mainly occurs in two regions under normal physiological conditions, the subventricular zone (SVZ) of the lateral ventricles and the subgranular zone (SGZ) of the hippocampal dentate gyrus [5, 6], where unique niche architectures permit continuous neurogenesis.

Moreover, it has been reported that neurogenesis occurs after stroke in the brain. Following an ischemic insult, the proliferation and/or dedifferentiation of endogenous neuronal stem cells is activated in various regions in the brain, including the SVZ, SGZ, striatum, and cerebral cortex [7], and these neuronal stem cells have been shown to migrate into the ischemic area, where neurogenesis does not occur under normal conditions [8–10]. Similar to the findings shown in the murine stroke model, we reported the presence of neural stem/progenitor cells in patients with stroke and that the peak of endogenous neurogenesis is approximately 1–2 weeks after a stroke [11]. These findings suggested the potential for a novel therapeutic strategy using stroke-induced neural stem/progenitor cells for neural function recovery in patients with stroke.

However, most of these stroke-induced neural stem/progenitor cells cannot survive, so they do not contribute to the functional recovery after stroke. Thus, appropriate support for the survival of these stroke-induced neural stem/progenitor cells is essential for functional recovery after cerebral ischemia.

12.3 Relationship Between Angiogenesis and Neurogenesis

Angiogenesis in the brain after stroke had been investigated as an important event for the survival of stroke-induced neural stem/progenitor cells and functional recovery. Recently, some reports suggested the tight correlation between angiogenesis and neurogenesis in adult songbirds [12] and in the premature mammalian brain [13]. Moreover, angiogenesis and neurogenesis are regulated by an overlapping set of molecules, such as sphingosine-1-phosphate, which plays a critical role in neurogenesis and angiogenesis during embryonic development [14]. These evidences indicate a close relationship between angiogenesis and neurogenesis in the brain. Therefore, we focused on therapeutic angiogenesis that could have an important role in the functional recovery of patients with stroke by enhancing neurogenesis in the poststroke brain [15] (Fig. 12.2).

12.4 Cell-Based Therapy to Enhance Neurogenesis in the Ischemic Brain

As an attractive cell source for angiogenesis in the ischemic tissue, bone marrow-derived mononuclear cells, a rich cell source of both hematopoietic stem cells and endothelial stem/progenitor cells, have been proposed. Previous reports suggested

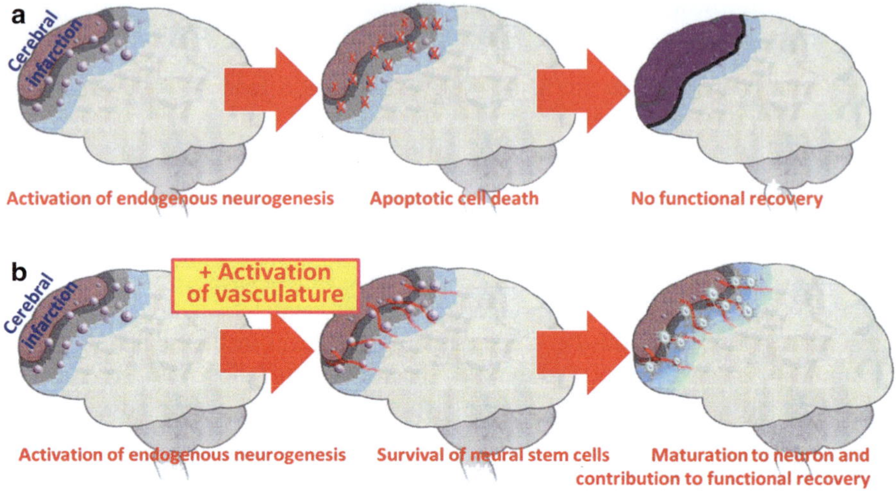

Fig. 12.2 Therapeutic angiogenesis enhances endogenous neurogenesis after stroke (Quoted and modified from [15]). Most of the stroke-induced neural stem cell cannot survive because of the unfavorable environments (**a**). Hematopoietic stem cell transplantation activates angiogenesis at the ischemia site and provides vascular niche for the survival of neural stem cells, followed by enhanced neurogenesis and functional recovery after stroke (**b**)

that endothelial stem/progenitor cells are key factors for maintaining vascular homeostasis and repair. Endothelial stem/progenitor cells have been shown to contribute to vascular homeostasis through differentiation into endothelial cells [16] and as a source of numerous growth and angiogenesis factors (e.g., vascular endothelial growth factor (VEGF), hepatocyte growth factor (HGF), and insulin-like growth factor I (IGF- I)) [17]. Endothelial stem/progenitor cells present in the bone marrow are effective for reducing ischemic damage and enhancing functional recovery in experimental models, including limb [18–21], myocardium [22–25], and cerebral ischemia [26, 27] models. Moreover, we observed that decreased levels of circulating immature bone marrow-derived cells in the peripheral blood are associated with impaired cerebrovascular function [27] and reduced cognitive function [28, 29]. On the other hand, high levels of bone marrow-derived immature cells are associated with neovascularization of the ischemic brain [30].

Based on these observations, a new strategy for enhancing neuronal regeneration in the brain after cerebral ischemia has been proposed. In a preclinical trial, we investigated the effect of administrating bone marrow-derived stem/progenitor cells for stroke using a highly reproducible murine model [31]. We evaluated the appropriate cell numbers and therapeutic time window for transplantation of bone marrow-derived mononuclear cells for patients with stroke. The results of this study indicated that the required minimum number of bone marrow-derived mononuclear cells was 1×10^6/kg of body weight and the therapeutic time window of cell therapy was between day 2 and day 14 after stroke [32]. This therapeutic time window was conformed to be the peak of endogenous neurogenesis after stroke [11]. These findings suggest that therapeutic strategy focused on angiogenesis using bone marrow mononuclear cells could become a novel cell therapy method for patients after stroke.

12.5 Phase 1/2a Clinical Trials Using Bone Marrow Mononuclear Cells in Patients After Stroke

Based on the findings of the preclinical trial, we conducted a clinical trial to enhance neurogenesis and functional recovery through activating angiogenesis using autologous bone marrow mononuclear cells for patients in the acute/subacute stroke stage. Our trial was an unblinded, uncontrolled phase 1/2a clinical trial. This clinical protocol was approved by the Ministry of Health, Labour and Welfare and the institutional review board of the National Cerebral and Cardiovascular Center (ClinicalTrials.gov Identifier: NCT01028794). The outline of this protocol is shown in Fig. 12.3. The aim of this clinical trial was to assess the feasibility, safety, and efficacy of intravenous transplantation of autologous bone marrow mononuclear cells into patients with stroke. Major inclusion criteria were patients with cerebral embolism, age 20–75 years, National Institute of Health Stroke Scale (NIHSS) score higher than 9 on day 7 after stroke, and NIHSS score displaying improvement of less than 6 points in the first 7 days after onset. On days 7–10 after stroke, patients had 25 mL (low-dose group, $N = 6$) or 50 mL (high-dose group, $N = 6$) of bone marrow cell aspiration from the posterior iliac bone under local anesthesia. Autologous bone marrow-derived mononuclear cells were purified by the density gradient method and administered intravenously on the same day as the aspiration. Primary outcome measures were worsening NIHSS score (primary safety outcome measure) and change in the NIHSS score evaluated on day 7 after onset of stroke and day 30 after cell transplantation (primary efficacy outcome measure). Secondary outcome measures were death at the time of discharge from the hospital (secondary safety outcome measure) and NIHSS score, modified Rankin scale (mRS) score, ratio of favorable outcome (defined as mRS ≤ 3), and Barthel Index score at days 30, 90, and 120 after cell transplantation (secondary efficacy outcome measures). We also evaluated the changes in the regional cerebral blood (rCBF) and regional cerebral metabolic rate of oxygen consumption ($rCMRO_2$) using steady-state ^{15}O positron emission tomography (PET) at 1 and 6 months after cell transplantation.

The results of this study showed that the transplantation of autologous bone marrow mononuclear cells in patients with severe stroke was feasible and safe. No side effects or safety problem was observed. Comparing the two doses (25 and 50 mL) of bone marrow mononuclear cells, the higher-dose treatment showed a positive trend compared with the lower-dose treatment (Fig. 12.4). Moreover, comparison to the historical control group also indicated significant better result in NIHSS by autologous bone marrow cell transplantation (Fig. 12.5). Most of the patients showed significantly improved function at 6 months after cell transplantation.

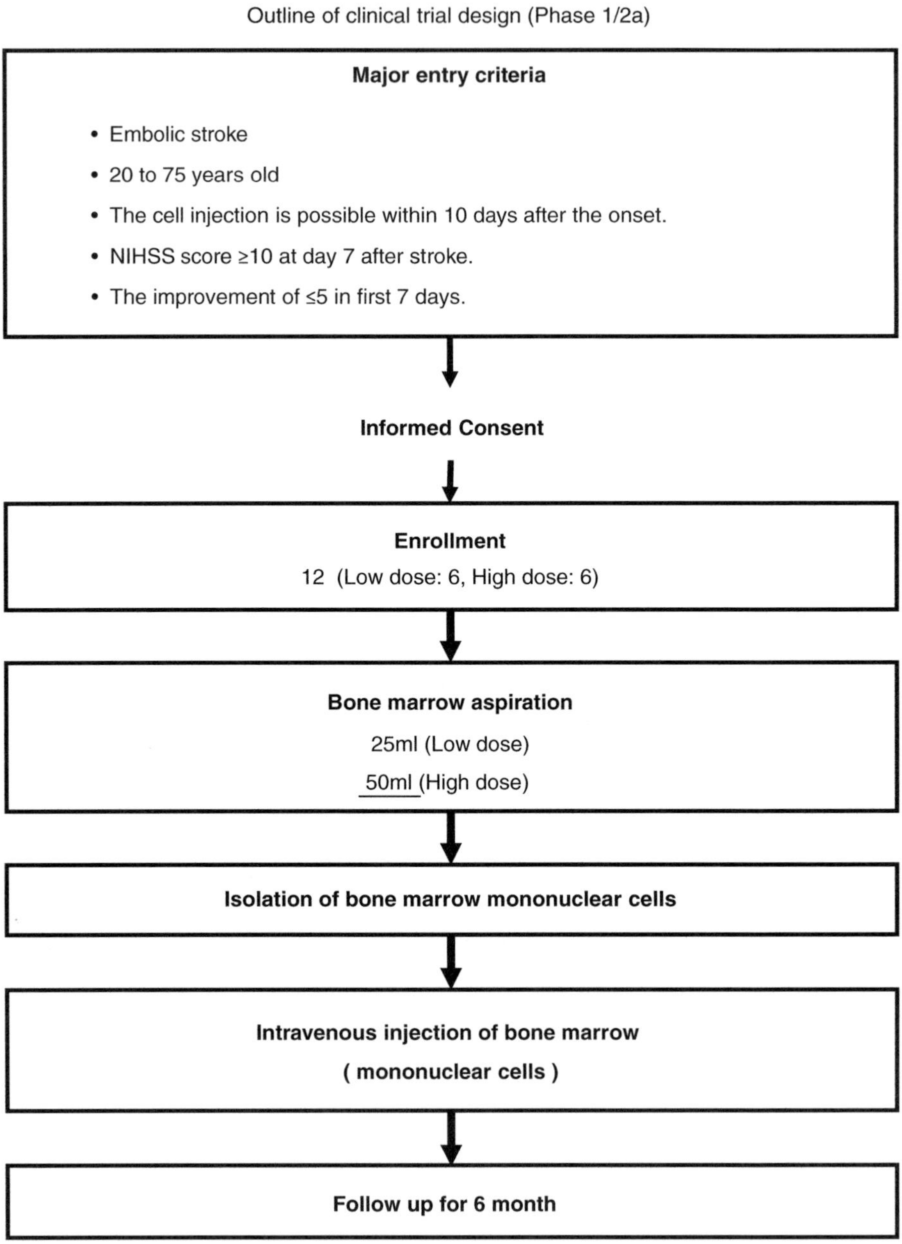

Fig. 12.3 Outline of clinical trial design (Quoted and modified from [33]). Our clinical trial was unblinded, uncontrolled phase 1/2a clinical trial. On 7–10 days after stroke, autologous bone marrow is aspirated. Isolation of bone marrow mononuclear cells and transplantation of bone marrow mononuclear cells are performed on the same day as the bone marrow aspiration

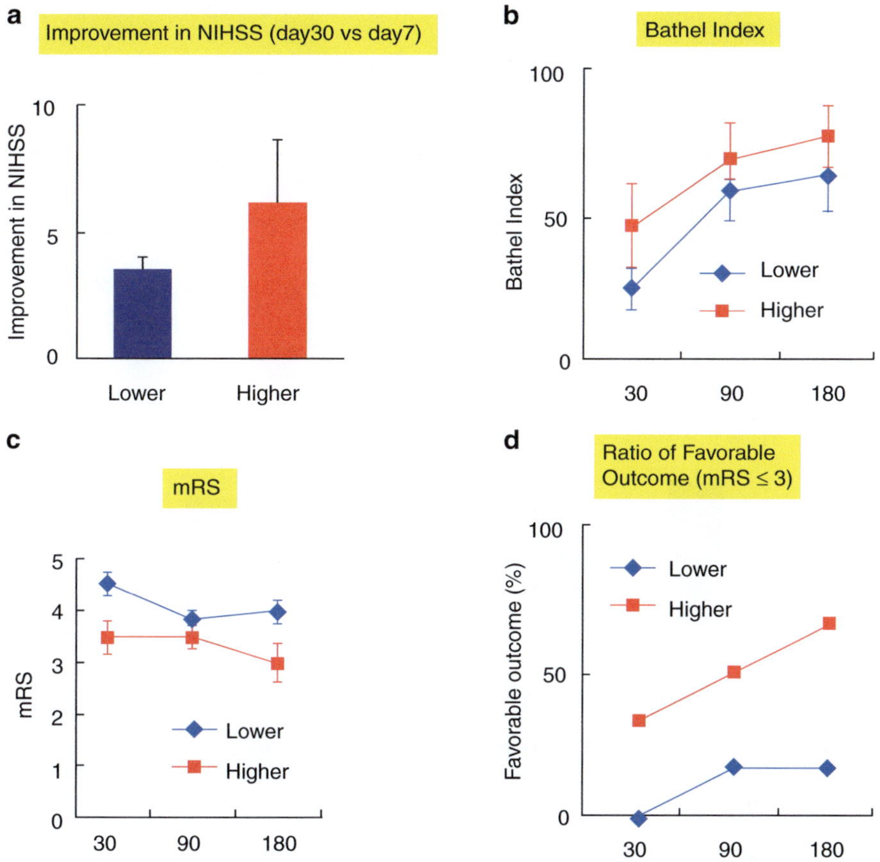

Fig. 12.4 Comparison of neurological outcomes between lower- and higher-dose group (Quoted and modified from [33]). Although there is no statistically significant difference in the improvement of NIHSS score (**a**), Barthel Index (**b**), mRS score (**c**), and ratio of favorable outcome (**d**) between groups, a clear trend toward improvement is observed in the higher-dose group in each case, compared with the lower-dose group

Furthermore, analysis of the cerebral blood flow and metabolism in patients after cell transplantation showed a trend favoring an increase in the rCBF and $rCMRO_2$ in both diseased and contralateral hemispheres at 6 months after cell transplantation, compared with 1 month. This clinical trial indicated that the autologous bone marrow mononuclear cell transplantation in patients with severe embolic stroke was feasible and safe. Furthermore, the positive trends showing effective neurologic recovery in a dose-dependent manner and improvement in cerebral blood flow and oxygen metabolism in poststroke patients after cell therapy emphasized the potential of this approach [33].

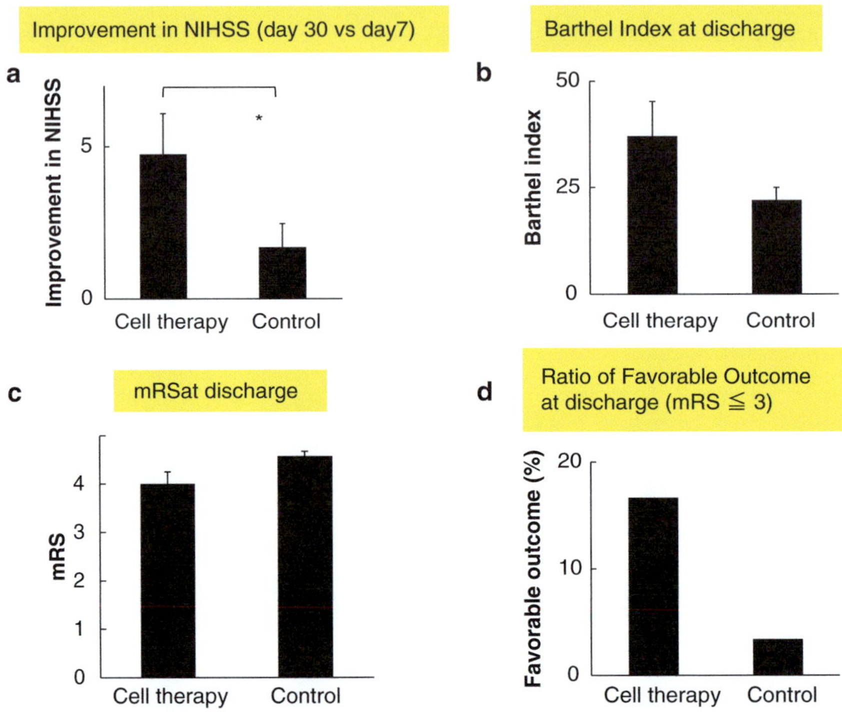

Fig. 12.5 Comparison of neurological outcomes between enrolled patients and historical controls at the time of discharge (Quoted and modified from [33]). Significant improvement of NIHSS score is observed in patients with cell transplantation (day 7 after onset of stroke vs. discharge) (**a**). Although there is no statistically significant difference in the Barthel Index (**b**), mRS score (**c**), and ratio of favorable outcome (**d**) between the groups, a clear trend toward improvement is observed in the cell therapy group in each case, compared with the historical controls

12.6 Regeneration Process and Other Cell Therapies After Stroke

We demonstrated that the transplantation of bone marrow-derived mononuclear cells in the subacute phase of stroke is effective for functional recovery in animal model and is feasible and safe in clinical trial [33]. These findings suggested that angiogenesis by bone marrow-derived stem/progenitor cells promoted neural and functional recovery in patients with stroke. We are planning the next phase of clinical trials to clearly prove the effect of this cell therapy.

In order to develop an effective stroke therapy, it is important to elucidate the regeneration process after stroke and optimize treatment methods. The regeneration process of wound healing is divided into the inflammatory phase of a few days after a failure (inflammatory phase) and subsequent growth phase for a few weeks (proliferative phase), followed by about 1 year of repair period (remodeling phase) (Fig. 12.6a), and it is known that optimization of each phase is important in wound

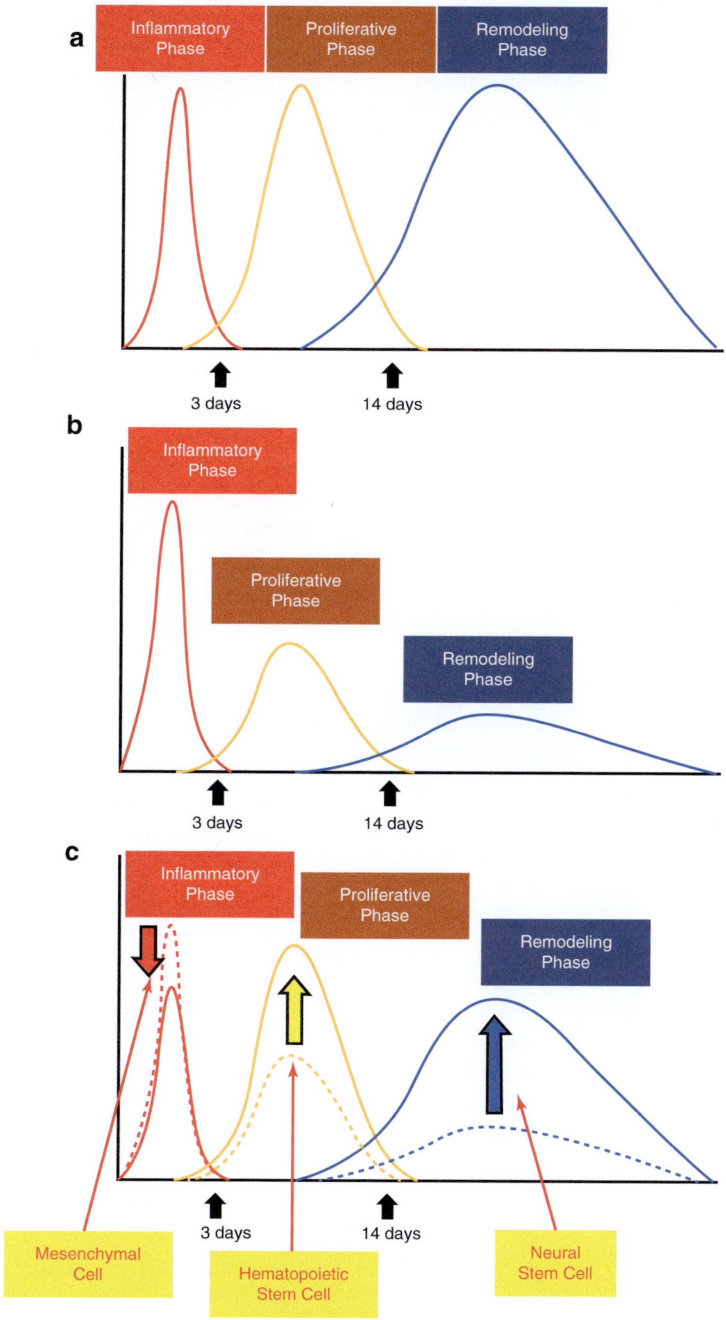

Fig. 12.6 Cell therapies and its targets (Quoted and modified from [15]). Although the regenerative processes are similar between skin injury (**a**) and stroke (**b**), the level of proliferative and remodeling phase is likely to be insufficient after stroke resulting in an incomplete functional recovery. Combination of each cell therapy and appropriate target has the potential to improve the regenerative process after stroke (**c**)

healing [34]. Similar to the regeneration process of wound healing, the regeneration process after stroke also consists of three phases, the acute phase of a few days immediately after stroke (inflammatory phase), the subacute phase after 2 weeks of stroke onset (growth phase), and the subsequent chronic phase (repair phase) (Fig.12.6b). Although we considered that the activation of angiogenesis in the growth phase is the most effective target for stroke therapy, other phases could also be targeted by regenerative medicine after stroke (Fig. 12.6c). The cell therapy in the inflammatory phase may be the target for the suppression of inflammation, i.e., using mesenchymal stem cells. Transplantation of allogeneic bone marrow-derived mesenchymal stem cells in the acute phase of stroke was performed in a clinical trial with a positive effect [35]. The importance of inhibition of excessive inflammatory responses in the acute stage of cerebral infarction has been suggested. In the remodeling phase of stroke, regeneration of neurons using neural stem cells has been considered. Some clinical trials for neural regeneration have been conducted, including transplantation of allogeneic teratocarcinoma-derived neuronal cells [3], fetal porcine-derived neural stem cells [4], human fetal neural stem cells [36], allogeneic mesenchymal-derived stem cells [35], and autologous mesenchymal stem cells [37]. Furthermore, recently, neural stem/progenitor cells derived from iPS cells have progressed basic research studies [38]. Based on these, neural stem cell transplantation may become the new cell therapy option in the remodeling phase of stroke.

In contrast, cell therapies that did not adhere to the appropriate time point did not show neural function recovery [32]. The optimal treatment in each phase would have maximum effect of functional recovery after stroke, and a combination of cell therapies in different phases can be one of the approaches for the best recovery of the adult brain from stroke in the future.

12.7 Conclusion

The findings obtained from basic research indicated that therapeutic angiogenesis by hematopoietic stem cell transplantation improves stroke outcomes through enhancing endogenous neurogenesis after stroke. The result obtained from clinical trial indicated that autologous bone marrow cell transplantation is safe and improves stroke outcomes. To further develop a more effective regenerative therapy for the adult brain, elucidation of the regeneration process and optimization of treatment for each phase after stroke are required.

References

1. Xu ZP, Li HH, Li YH, Zhang Y, Wu Q, Lin L. Feasibility and outcomes of intravenous thrombolysis 3–4.5 hours after stroke in Chinese patients. J Clin Neurosci. 2014;21:822–6.
2. Kasahara Y, Matsuyama T, Taguchi A. Treatment of autologous bone marrow mononuclear cells for acute and subacute stroke. In: Hess DC, editor. Cell therapy for brain injury. Switzerland: Springer; 2015. p. 37–46.

3. Kondziolka D, Wechsler L, Goldstein S, Meltzer C, Thulborn KR, Gebel J, et al. Transplantation of cultured human neuronal cells for patients with stroke. Neurology. 2000;55:565–9.
4. Savitz SI, Dinsmore J, Wu J, Henderson GV, Stieg P, Caplan LR. Neurotransplantation of fetal porcine cells in patients with basal ganglia infarcts: a preliminary safety and feasibility study. Cerebrovasc Dis. 2005;20:101–7.
5. Lledo PM, Alonso M, Grubb MS. Adult neurogenesis and functional plasticity in neuronal circuits. Nat Rev Neurosci. 2006;7:179–93.
6. Ma DK, Bonaguidi MA, Ming GL, Song H. Adult neural stem cells in the mammalian central nervous system. Cell Res. 2009;19:672–82.
7. Darsalia V, Heldmann U, Lindvall O, Kokaia Z. Stroke-induced neurogenesis in aged brain. Stroke. 2005;36:1790–5.
8. Arvidsson A, Collin T, Kirik D, Kokaia Z, Lindvall O. Neuronal replacement from endogenous precursors in the adult brain after stroke. Nat Med. 2002;8:963–70.
9. Parent JM, Vexler ZS, Gong C, Derugin N, Ferriero DM. Rat forebrain neurogenesis and striatal neuron replacement after focal stroke. Ann Neurol. 2002;52:802–13.
10. Zhang R, Zhang Z, Wang L, Wang Y, Gousev A, Zhang L, et al. Activated neural stem cells contribute to stroke-induced neurogenesis and neuroblast migration toward the infarct boundary in adult rats. J Cereb Blood Flow Metab. 2004;24:441–8.
11. Nakayama D, Matsuyama T, Ishibashi-Ueda H, Nakagomi T, Kasahara Y, Hirose H, et al. Injury-induced neural stem/progenitor cells in post-stroke human cerebral cortex. Eur J Neurosci. 2010;31:90–8.
12. Louissaint A Jr, Rao S, Leventhal C, Goldman SA. Coordinated interaction of neurogenesis and angiogenesis in the adult songbird brain. Neuron. 2002;34:945–60.
13. Shin HY, Kim JH, Phi JH, Park CK, Kim JE, Kim JH, et al. Endogenous neurogenesis and neovascularization in the neocortex of the rat after focal cerebral ischemia. J Neurosci Res. 2008;86:356–67.
14. Mizugishi K, Yamashita T, Olivera A, Miller GF, Spiegel S, Proia RL. Essential role for sphingosine kinases in neural and vascular development. Mol Cell Biol. 2005;25:11113–21.
15. Taguchi A. Cell-based therapy for stroke patients. No Sinkei Geka. 2015;43:1071–9.
16. Asahara T, Murohara T, Sullivan A, Silver M, van der Zee R, Li T, et al. Isolation of putative progenitor endothelial cells for angiogenesis. Science. 1997;275:964–7.
17. Majka M, Janowska-Wieczorek A, Ratajczak J, Ehrenman K, Pietrzkowski Z, Kowalska MA, et al. Numerous growth factors, cytokines, and chemokines are secreted by human CD34(+) cells, myeloblasts, erythroblasts, and megakaryoblasts and regulate normal hematopoiesis in an autocrine/paracrine manner. Blood. 2001;97:3075–85.
18. Duong Van Huyen JP, Smadja DM, Bruneval P, Gaussem P, Dal-Cortivo L, Julia P, et al. Bone marrow-derived mononuclear cell therapy induces distal angiogenesis after local injection in critical leg ischemia. Mod Pathol. 2008;21:837–46.
19. Tachi Y, Fukui D, Wada Y, Koshikawa M, Shimodaira S, Ikeda U, et al. Changes in angiogenesis-related factors in serum following autologous bone marrow cell implantation for severe limb ischemia. Expert Opin Biol Ther. 2008;8:705–12.
20. Talapkova R, Hudecek J, Sinak I, Kubisz P, Laca L, Hlinka L, et al. The salvage of ischaemic limb by therapeutical angiogenesis. Vnitr Lek. 2009;55:179–83.
21. Padilla L, Krotzsch E, De La Garza AS, Figueroa S, Rodriguez-Trejo J, Avila G, et al. Bone marrow mononuclear cells stimulate angiogenesis when transplanted into surgically induced fibrocollagenous tunnels: results from a canine ischemic hindlimb model. Microsurgery. 2007;27:91–7.
22. Tatsumi T, Matsubara H. Therapeutic angiogenesis for peripheral arterial disease and ischemic heart disease by autologous bone marrow cells implantation. Nippon Rinsho. 2006;64:2126–34.
23. Tse HF, Siu CW, Zhu SG, Songyan L, Zhang QY, Lai WH, et al. Paracrine effects of direct intramyocardial implantation of bone marrow derived cells to enhance neovascularization in chronic ischaemic myocardium. Eur J Heart Fail. 2007;9:747–53.
24. Yokokura Y, Hayashida N, Okazaki T, Nakamura E, Tayama E, Akashi H, et al. Influence of angiogenesis by implantation of bone marrow mononuclear cells in the rat ischemic heart. Kurume Med J. 2007;54:77–84.

25. Zen K, Okigaki M, Hosokawa Y, Adachi Y, Nozawa Y, Takamiya M, et al. Myocardium-targeted delivery of endothelial progenitor cells by ultrasound-mediated microbubble destruction improves cardiac function via an angiogenic response. J Mol Cell Cardiol. 2006;40:799–809.
26. Fan Y, Shen F, Frenzel T, Zhu W, Ye J, Liu J, et al. Endothelial progenitor cell transplantation improves long-term stroke outcome in mice. Ann Neurol. 2010;67:488–97.
27. Taguchi A, Matsuyama T, Moriwaki H, Hayashi T, Hayashida K, Nagatsuka K, et al. Circulating CD34-positive cells provide an index of cerebrovascular function. Circulation. 2004;109:2972–5.
28. Taguchi A, Matsuyama T, Nakagomi T, Shimizu Y, Fukunaga R, Tatsumi Y, et al. Circulating CD34-positive cells provide a marker of vascular risk associated with cognitive impairment. J Cereb Blood Flow Metab. 2008;28:445–9.
29. Taguchi A, Nakagomi N, Matsuyama T, Kikuchi-Taura A, Yoshikawa H, Kasahara Y, et al. Circulating CD34-positive cells have prognostic value for neurologic function in patients with past cerebral infarction. J Cereb Blood Flow Metab. 2009;29:34–8.
30. Yoshihara T, Taguchi A, Matsuyama T, Shimizu Y, Kikuchi-Taura A, Soma T, et al. Increase in circulating CD34-positive cells in patients with angiographic evidence of moyamoya-like vessels. J Cereb Blood Flow Metab. 2008;28:1086–9.
31. Taguchi A, Kasahara Y, Nakagomi T, Stern DM, Fukunaga M, Ishikawa M, et al. A reproducible and simple model of permanent cerebral ischemia in CB-17 and SCID mice. J Exp Stroke Transl Med. 2010;3:28–33.
32. Uemura M, Kasahara Y, Nagatsuka K, Taguchi A. Cell-based therapy to promote angiogenesis in the brain following ischemic damage. Curr Vasc Pharmacol. 2012;10:285–8.
33. Taguchi A, Sakai C, Soma T, Kasahara Y, Stern DM, Kajimoto K, et al. Intravenous autologous bone marrow mononuclear cell transplantation for stroke: Phase1/2a clinical trial in a homogeneous group of stroke patients. Stem Cells Dev. 2015;24:2207–18.
34. Reinke JM, Sorg H. Wound repair and regeneration. Eur Surg Res. 2012;49:35–43.
35. Hess DC, Hill WD, Martin-Studdard A, Carroll J, Brailer J, Carothers J. Bone marrow as a source of endothelial cells and NeuN-expressing cells after stroke. Stroke. 2002;33:1362–8.
36. Hassani Z, O'Reilly J, Pearse Y, Stroemer P, Tang E, Sinden J, et al. Human neural progenitor cell engraftment increases neurogenesis and microglial recruitment in the brain of rats with stroke. PLoS One. 2012;7:e50444.
37. Honmou O, Houkin K, Matsunaga T, Niitsu Y, Ishiai S, Onodera R, et al. Intravenous administration of auto serum-expanded autologous mesenchymal stem cells in stroke. Brain. 2011;134:1790–807.
38. Oki K, Tatarishvili J, Wood J, Koch P, Wattananit S, Mine Y, et al. Human-induced pluripotent stem cells form functional neurons and improve recovery after grafting in stroke-damaged brain. Stem Cells. 2012;30:1120–33.

Chapter 13
Clinical Trials on Cell Therapy for Perinatal Brain Injury: Challenges and Opportunities

Noriko Takahashi and Rintaro Mori

Abstract We performed a review of the literature and identified 9 published studies that conducted clinical trials to identify the safety, feasibility, and efficacy of cell therapy and 16 ongoing clinical trials. Most studies showed an improvement of motor function compared to the control groups, and the improvement appeared in the relatively early stage after transplantation. However, the mechanism by which stem cells help to recover neurological cells remains unclear. Many of the studies or trials were in phase 1 or phase 2; thus, it is too early to conclude the effectiveness of cell therapy. Therefore, further clinical trials at an advanced stage and experimental research using animal models are needed to elucidate the mechanism and efficacy. Conversely, the pharmaceutical agencies that review new drugs and medical devices have installed various systems and policies to accelerate the development of new drugs. For instance, the Pharmaceuticals and Medical Devices Agency (PMDA) has established a special department for cellular and tissue-based products; furthermore, the PMDA has launched a conditional time-limited marketing authorization system. This system makes it possible to rapidly provide new drugs to patients. In addition, the PMDA has installed an accelerated assessment system to facilitate the development of drugs for diseases without route-based treatment.

Keywords Clinical trial · Review · PMDA

13.1 Clinical Trials with Cell Therapy for Pediatric Brain Injury

13.1.1 Current Trials for Children

Although many clinical trials to investigate the efficacy and feasibility of the cell therapy against pediatric brain injury have been registered, the number of published research is low [1–16]. As a result of an electronic database search using the retrieve

N. Takahashi, Ph.D. • R. Mori, M.D., Ph.D. (✉)
Department of Health Policy, National Center for Child Health and Development, Tokyo, Japan
e-mail: rintaromori@gmail.com

© Springer Nature Singapore Pte Ltd. 2018

H. Shintaku et al. (eds.), *Cell Therapy for Perinatal Brain Injury*,
https://doi.org/10.1007/978-981-10-1412-3_13

Table 13.1 Published studies using cell therapy

	Author	Study title	Year	Results
1	Hassan et al. [22]	Stem cell transplantation in Egyptian patients with cerebral palsy	2012	Highly significant improvement on motor, independence, and communication skills
2	Luan et al. [20]	Effects of neural progenitor cell transplantation in children with severe cerebral palsy	2012	Significant improvement of motor function 1 month after transplantation. Greater improvement was observed in all tests
3	Chen et al. [17]	Neural stem cell-like cells derived from autologous bone mesenchymal stem cells for the treatment of patients with cerebral palsy	2013	Optimal improvement of motor function 3 months after transplantation. No improvement on language function
4	Luan et al. [21]	Neural stem/progenitor cell transplantation for cortical visual impairment in neonatal brain-injured patients	2013	Effective for treating children with severe visual impairment; however, in some cases, the effectiveness was low
5	Min et al. [24]	Umbilical cord blood therapy potentiated with erythropoietin for children with cerebral palsy: A double-blind, randomized, placebo-controlled trial	2013	Significantly higher scores on the GMPM and BSID-II mental and motor scales at 6 months. Structural and metabolic changes in the brain were observed
6	Wang et al. [25]	Effects of bone marrow mesenchymal stromal cells on gross motor function measure scores of children with cerebral palsy	2013	Total score improved at 1, 6, and 18 months after transplantation compared to the baseline score. The fastest motor function recovery occurred within 3–6 months but gradually slowed
7	Cotton et al. [18]	Feasibility of autologous cord blood cells for infants with hypoxic-ischemic encephalopathy	2014	Mortality was not statistically significant. Regarding vital signs, cell recipients, and concurrent cooled infants had similar hospital outcomes. Thirteen of 18 (74%) cell recipients and 19 of 46 (41%) concurrent cooled infants with known 1-year outcomes survived with Bayley scores ≥85
8	Mancias-Guerra et al. [23]	Safety and tolerability of intrathecal delivery of autologous bone marrow nucleated cells in children with CP: open-labeled phase 1 trial	2014	Bone marrow stimulation and harvesting were observed. However, no change was found in MRI
9	Kang et al. [19]	Involvement of immune responses in the efficacy of cord blood cell therapy for CP	2015	Greater improvement on muscle strength and motor outcomes. Induced systemic immune reactions and anti-inflammatory changes were observed

style, the nine articles shown in Table 13.1 were identified [17–25]. Of these, the clinical target of eight studies was pediatric cerebral palsy (CP) in infants, and the remaining study was on hypoxic-ischemic encephalopathy (HIE) in neonates [17–25]. The age of the subjects varied widely, from 1 month to 20 years of age, although all the trials targeted pediatric patients [17–25].

The stem cells used for the trials were derived from the bone marrow or umbilical cord blood (UCB). In the studies, bone marrow-derived stem cells were frequently used for cell therapy; however, current research using stem cells derived from UCB is being performed in the ongoing trials shown in Table 13.2 [1–16]. Improvements were observed in all studies, and the most remarkable improvement occurred in motor and visual functions [17, 19–22, 24, 25]. Some studies showed an improvement in the motor function early after stem cell transplantation [17, 25]. Furthermore, an improvement appeared as early as 1 month after transplantation in one study [20]. Conversely, some studies have reported that a significant improvement was not observed in the mortality or language ability [17]. Only two studies were double-blinded, and one study was open-labeled observer-blinded [17, 19, 24]. The remaining studies were non-blinded.

13.1.2 Ongoing Research

A number of clinical trials have been conducted worldwide, and we identified 16 ongoing clinical trials using cell therapy in neonates or infants with various types of brain diseases [1–16]. Among these cases, only one phase 3 trial is currently being conducted [1], while the other ones are still in phase 1 or phase 2 [2–7, 9–16]. Although most previously published studies targeted infants older than 1 years of age, six of the ongoing trials target neonates [3, 5, 13–16]. Of these, the age target of four trials is within 24 h [3, 14–16], with the two remaining studies within 14 days after birth [5, 13]. The ongoing trials are being conducted in the USA and Asian countries; seven trials have been carried out in the USA [2–6, 11, 12], and the other studies have been carried out in the Republic of Korea, China, Japan, and Singapore [1, 7–10, 13–16]. No ongoing trial has been carried out in European countries. No results are available thus far; however, further results that promote cell therapy for pediatric brain injury are anticipated in the near future. As mentioned in 13-1-1, UCB infusion is becoming the major treatment for cell therapy in neonates or infants in the ongoing clinical trials. Furthermore, most trials have adopted autologous stem cells that have a lower rejection response, suggesting that additional research using autologous UCB may be actively conducted in the future.

13.1.3 Challenge of Future Studies

Although a number of published studies and ongoing clinical trials have been registered, the sample size was small. The number of subjects in the intervention groups varied from 17 to 46, and the control groups had similar numbers of subjects

Table 13.2 Ongoing clinical trials for pediatric brain injury using cell therapy

	ID number	Title	Institution	Clinical target	Intervention
1	NCT00593242 [5]	Cord Blood for Neonatal Hypoxic-Ischemic Encephalopathy	Duke University Medical Center, USA	Neonatal hypoxic-ischemic encephalopathy	Autologous umbilical cord blood
2	NCT01649648 [13]	Autologous Cord Blood Cells for Brain Injury in Term Newborns	National University Hospital, Singapore	Hypoxic-ischemic encephalopathy	Autologous umbilical cord blood
3	NCT01072370 [4]	Safety and Effectiveness of Cord Blood Stem Cell Infusion for the Treatment of Cerebral Palsy in Children	Georgia Regents University, USA	Cerebral palsy	Cord blood
4	NCT01147653 [11]	A Randomized Study of Autologous Umbilical Cord Blood Reinfusion in Children With Cerebral Palsy	Duke University Medical Center, USA	Cerebral palsy	Autologous umbilical cord blood
5	NCT01769716 [9]	Umbilical Cord Blood Therapy for Global Developmental Delay	Bundang CHA Hospital, Republic of Korea	Global developmental delay	Allogenic/autologous umbilical cord blood
6	NCT01885663 [10]	UCB Therapy in Acquired Brain Injury	Bundang CHA Hospital, Republic of Korea	Acquired brain injury	Umbilical cord blood
7	NCT01884155 [7]	Allogeneic Umbilical Cord Blood Therapy for Stroke	Bundang CHA Hospital, Republic of Korea	Stroke	Allogeneic umbilical cord blood
8	NCT01929434 [1]	Efficacy of Stem Cell Transplantation Compared to Rehabilitation Treatment of Patients With Cerebral Paralysis (CP)	General Hospital of Chinese Armed Police Forces, China	Cerebral paralysis	Stem cells
9	NCT01988584 [6]	Safety and Effectiveness of Banked Cord Blood or Bone Morrow Stem Cells in Children With Cerebral Palsy (CP) (ACT for CP)	The University of Texas Health Science Center, USA	Cerebral palsy	Autologous stem cells
10	NCT02025972 [8]	Allogeneic Umbilical Cord Blood Therapy in Children With CP	Bundang CHA Hospital, Republic of Korea	Cerebral palsy	Allogeneic umbilical cord blood
11	NCT02256618 [14]	Autologous Cord Blood Cell Therapy for Neonatal Encephalopathy	Neonatal Encephalopathy Consortium, Japan	Neonatal encephalopathy Hypoxic-ischemic encephalopathy	Autologous umbilical cord blood

	ID number	Title	Institution	Clinical target	Intervention
12	NCT02434965 [3]	Autologous Cord Blood and Human Placental Derived Stem Cells in Neonates With Severe Hypoxic-Ischemic Encephalopathy (HPDSC + HIE)	New York Medical College, USA	Severe hypoxic-ischemic encephalopathy	Human placental-derived stem cells (HPDSC) in combination with autologous umbilical cord blood
13	NCT02460484 [2]	Safety of Autologous Human Umbilical Cord Blood Treatment For Perinatal Arterial Ischemic Stroke	Florida Hospital, USA	Perinatal arterial ischemic stroke	Autologous umbilical cord blood
14	NCT02551003 [16]	Neuroprotective Effect Of Autologous Cord Blood Combined With Therapeutic Hypothermia Following Neonatal Encephalopathy	Children's Hospital of Fudan University, China	Hypoxic-ischemic encephalopathy Cerebral infarction	Autologous umbilical cord blood
15	NCT02599207 [12]	Assessment of the Safety of Allogeneic Umbilical Cord Blood Infusions in Children With Cerebral Palsy	Duke University Medical Center, USA	Cerebral palsy	Sibling umbilical cord blood
16	NCT02605018 [15]	Neuroprotective Effect of Autologous Cord Blood Combined With Therapeutic Hypothermia Following Neonatal Encephalopathy	The People's Hospital of Dehong Autonomous Prefecture, China	Hypoxic-ischemic encephalopathy Cerebral infarction	Autologous umbilical cord blood

[17–25]. The follow-up period, moreover, was relatively short, and most studies followed the patients for 6 months to 1 year after finishing their treatment [17–20, 22–24]. Thus, the follow-up period was fewer than 2 years. In some cases, it was difficult to follow the patients because the patients lived thousands of miles away from the hospital where they received the treatment [18]. Accordingly, it is difficult to comprehensively judge whether cell therapy is efficient for infants or neonates with brain injury at this stage.

Because most studies remain in phase 1 or phase 2, the sample size might be small, and the follow-up periods might be relatively short. However, it is necessary for future clinical trials to include larger sample sizes and longer follow-up periods to precisely assess the efficacy and long-term effect of cell therapy. Many of the current clinical trials have been open-label because of their phase, although the implementation of more double-blinded clinical trials to determine the effectiveness of treatment is greatly needed.

Some animal research has also stated that treatment using UCB is beneficial for rodents with acute neonatal hypoxic-ischemic encephalopathy; however, the mechanism by which stem cells improve neurologic impairment remains unclear [26–28]. As with clinical trials, further experimental research using animal models is needed to elucidate the mechanism.

Bone marrow- or UCB-derived stem cells have been used as treatment in the previous studies and/or ongoing clinical trials. The types of stem cell differed in each study; for instance, Mancias-Guerra et al. used bone marrow-derived total nucleated cells. Conversely, Chen et al. used bone marrow-derived neural stem cell-like cells [17]. The timing of stem cell infusion or the amount of stem cells also differed in each study. In future studies, it is essential to verify the optimal combination of cell therapy and timing of infusing cells. Additionally, it is necessary to consider whether single or multiple transplantation is sufficient to recover neurological cells.

Regarding the outcome measurement, various scales to measure the motor function are used; however, more advanced and specific methods are needed to detect structural or functional changes.

13.2 Overview of the Review for Drugs and Medical Devices

13.2.1 Regulatory Authorities

In Japan, the Ministry of Health, Labour and Welfare (MHLW) and Pharmaceuticals and Medical Devices Agency (PMDA) are involved in reviewing drugs, medical devices, and cellular and tissue-based products (CTPs) [29, 30]. While the MHLW is concerned with legal issues, such as the establishment or revision of law regarding medical products, the PMDA reviews and approves new drugs, medical devices, and CTPs. Moreover, the PMDA leads the establishment of pharmaceutical regulations worldwide, alongside the US Food and Drug Administration (FDA) and European Medical Agency (EMA) [31, 32]. The guidelines regarding the development of medical products among the USA, European Union (EU), and Japan are determined in the International Conference on Harmonization of Technical Requirements for Registration of Pharmaceuticals for Human Use (ICH) [33]. The development of medical products in each country is controlled according to these guidelines.

13.2.2 Approach of the PMDA to Accelerate the Development of Cellular and Tissue-Based Products

13.2.2.1 Establishment of a New Framework

CTPs are made from human cells, implying that they may vary among different individuals. Hence, the quality of CTPs is likely to be inhomogeneous, and approvals for CTPs require more time than those for drugs or medical devices [29, 30]. Furthermore, a specialized department for CTPs was not established by the PMDA; thus it currently takes a substantial amount of time to provide CTPs to patients. The MHLW and PMDA, however, have embarked to take measures to solve the above situation. Only two frameworks of the medical products previously existed: drugs and medical devices. For this reason, CTPs were reviewed under medical devices. The PMDA recently established a specialized department for CTPs in order to be able to rapidly provide CTPs to patients.

13.2.2.2 The Revision of Laws and Installation of the New Approval System

It is time-consuming to develop a new drug because there are several steps before regulatory submission. Drug manufacturers generally spend 2–3 years on basic research and 3–5 years on non-clinical testing, as shown in Fig. 13.1. They also spend an additional 3–7 years on clinical trials. The regulatory authority of each country has attempted to shorten the review period in order to provide innovative drugs to patients as rapidly as possible.

The MHLW has officially announced two revised laws to promote CTPs and rapidly provide drugs and medical devices to patients. The first law is the Act on the Safety of Regenerative Medicine [29]. This law allows medical institutions to outsource cell cultures and processing cells, thus being able to rapidly provide CTPs to patients. The second law is the Revised Japanese Pharmaceutical Law [29]. This conditional time-limited marketing authorization system was implemented to introduce newly developed medical products on the market early (Fig. 13.2). The drug manufacturers were previously mandated to complete phase 3 clinical trials and gain all relevant data prior to regulatory submission. However, in the newly revised system, given that efficacy and safety of the medical products are demonstrated in phase 2 trials, the drug manufacturers can apply for regulatory submission, even without the completion of phase 3 trials. Conditional time-limited marketing

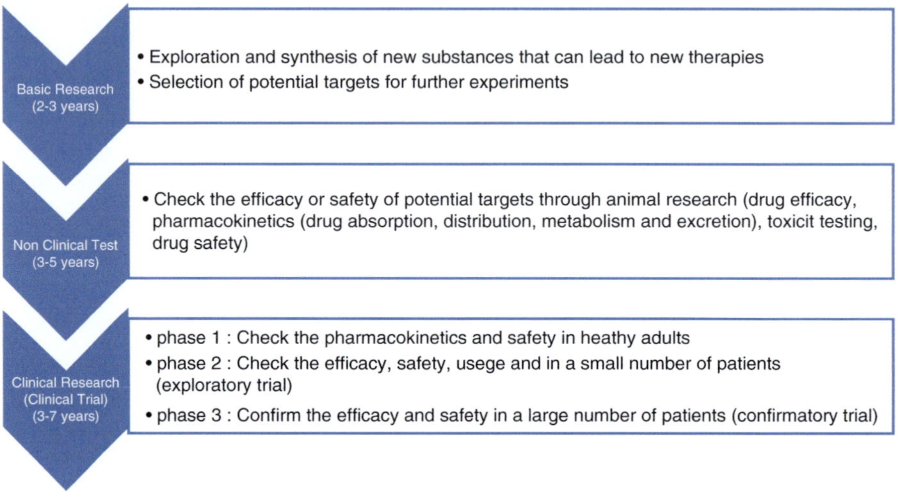

Fig. 13.1 Steps for drug development. This figure demonstrates the flow of drug development from the initial stage to clinical trials of drug development. The figure shows the content of each stage and approximate duration for each stage

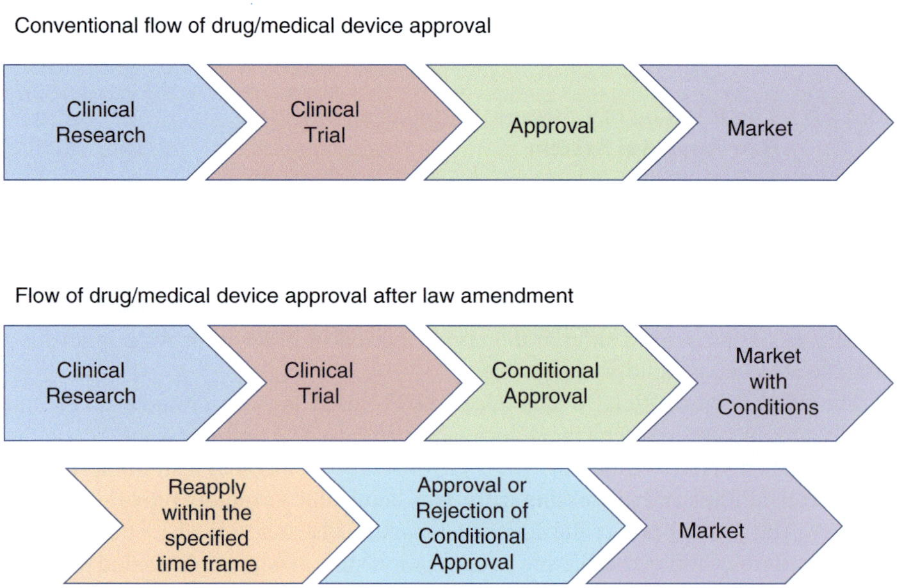

Fig. 13.2 Flow of drug and medical device review. This figure demonstrates the flow of the conventional and newly installed approved systems for the development of new drugs and medical devices

authorization will be given to the medical products that pass through the review, and the products can appear on the market with conditions. The drug manufacturers, however, must complete the phase 3 trials and obtain necessary data to reapply within a specified period. The products that are resubmitted within the appointed period are reviewed again, and it is determined whether the products are suitable to be given to patients. When the medical products passed the reviews, the drug manufacturers can continue to provide them to patients.

The MHLW has also instructed the drug manufacturers, clinical practice, and the PMDA to take considerable safety measures when introducing the conditional approval system. For clinical practice, clinicians must attempt to provide appropriate explanations to patients and obtain their informed consent. For the drug manufacturers, they have to keep records for post-marketing safety measures. For the PMDA, when patients suffer from health hazards due to the use of CTPs, they have to be rescued by the Relief Services for Adverse Health Effects.

13.2.2.3 Installation of the Accelerated Assessment System

The PMDA has introduced an accelerated assessment system and divided medical products into two priorities: priority review products and ordinary review products [30].

To apply for the accelerated assessment system, the medical products must fulfill the following items:

1. The medical products must exhibit new action mechanisms.
2. The medical products must be used for diseases that can seriously damage human life or diseases without route-based treatments.
3. The medical products must exhibit a high efficacy against the diseases as compared to existing drugs, or there are no current drugs for the diseases.
4. The medical products must initially be developed in Japan and be applied first in Japan.

Once the medical products are designated as priority products, specific reviewers from the PMDA are selected. The reviewers work closely with relevant departments of the MHLW and control the process of the development of the medical products, which makes it possible to develop medical products rapidly.

13.2.3 The Trend of Foreign Countries Regarding Cellular and Tissue-Based Products

13.2.3.1 Handling of Cellular and Tissue-Based Products

Handling of CTPs differs by countries. For instance, Japan has set up the department of CTPs for regulatory submission, and all products related to CTPs are reviewed by this department. However, when CTPs are used for clinical studies, regulatory submission is not necessary.

Table 13.3 Handling of cellular and tissue-based products in each country

Country/region	Regulatory authority	Classification of handling of cellular and tissue-based products	Review department
Japan	PMDA	• Cellular and tissue-based products	Department of Cellular and Tissue-based Products
USA	FDA	• Biologics (Primary mode of action is biochemical, immunological, or metabolic function)	Center for Biologics Evaluation and Research (CBER)
		• Medical devices (Primary mode of action is physical or structural function)	Center for Devices and Radiological Health (CDRH)
EU	EMA	• Advanced therapy medical products (ATMP) –Tissue therapy –Cell therapy –Gene therapy	Committee for Advanced Therapies (CAT)

Conversely, the US FDA announced the human cell, tissue, and cellular and tissue-based product under Section 351 or 361 that mentioned handling of CTPs [31]. According to the 351 HCT/P, CTPs are divided into the following two frameworks according to the primary mode of action: biologics or medical devices (Table 13.3). When using the biochemical, immunological, or metabolic function of cells or tissues, the products are sorted as biologics and must be applied to the FDA as biologics. When the physical or structural function is used for the products, they are regulated as medical devices. In the USA, all studies or trials that use CTPs are regulated by the same rule; thus all facilities that use CTPs require registration, suitable donor selection, and quality control [31].

In EU countries, gene therapy and cell therapy are evaluated as advanced therapy medical products (ATMPs) [32]. ATMPs are classified into the following three divisions: tissue therapy, cell therapy, and gene therapy. The products with biochemical, immunological, and metabolic functions are classified as tissue therapy, and the products using the physical or structural function of cells or tissues are reviewed as cell therapy. ATMPs are reviewed by the Committee for Advanced Therapies (CAT) because more exclusive and multidiscipline knowledge are needed [32]. The CAT is established under the Committee for Medical Products for Human Use (CHMP) and assesses the quality, safety, and efficacy of ATMPs [32].

13.2.3.2 The Early Approval System

The FDA previously introduced the following four approaches to increase the availability of new drugs in the early 1990s: (1) priority review, (2) breakthrough therapy, (3) accelerated approval, and (4) fast track [31]. These approaches apply for drugs that are the first treatment for diseases or are highly advantageous over existing drugs.

The priority review was installed in 1992 to improve the turnover time of drug review, and a two-tiered system to reduce the review time has been created: the priority review and standard review. The FDA's goal in the priority review is to take action on an application within 6 months. The breakthrough system is a process to facilitate the development and review of drugs that show a substantial improvement over the existing treatment. The FDA instituted the Accelerated Approval regulations in 1992. These regulations allow drugs that fulfill an unmet medical need to be approved in accordance with the results of a surrogated endpoint. Fast track is a process to facilitate the development and review of drugs that fulfill an unmet medical need. The fast track system applies for a wide spectrum of serious conditions.

The EMA has recently revised the guideline on the implementation of the accelerated assessment and conditional marketing authorization systems [32]. Both systems were installed to develop innovative medicines that target diseases without any effective treatment or medicines that may demonstrate substantial effects over existing drugs. The revised guideline makes it possible to optimize the assessment schedule and start early dialog with the EMA to facilitate the development and accelerated assessment of innovative medicine. Furthermore, the guideline presents information on conditional marketing authorization that allows for the early approval of medicines according to less complete clinical data. However, the available data must demonstrate that the benefits of public health outweigh its risks, and comprehensive clinical data should be obtained after authorization within a timeframe agreed upon with the CMPH.

13.3 Conclusion

Although many clinical trials have been conducted to identify the safety or feasibility of cell therapy for pediatric brain injury, the research is still in progress. Therefore, it is not easy to determine the efficacy of cell therapy at this stage. The implementation of more clinical trials at an advanced stage is necessary to gain benefits from the clinical trials in the future. Conversely, the pharmaceutical regulatory agencies of several countries have attempted to shorten the review time and facilitate the development of cell therapy by establishing new policies and systems. This contributes to the early application of medical products to patients.

References

1. An Y. Efficacy of stem cell transplantation compared to rehabilitation treatment of patients with cerebral paralysis (CP). 2013–2015. https://clinicaltrials.gov/ct2/show/NCT01929434?term=NCT01929434&rank=1. Accessed 30 Nov 2015.
2. Baumgartner J. Safety of autologous human umbilical cord blood treatment for perinatal arterial ischemic stroke. 2015–2019. https://clinicaltrials.gov/ct2/show/NCT02460484?term=NCT02460484&rank=1. Accessed 30 Nov 2015.

3. Cairo SM. Autologous cord blood and human placental derived stem cells in neonates with severe hypoxic-ischemic encephalopathy (HPDSC+HIE). 2016–2019. https://clinicaltrials.gov/ct2/show/NCT02434965?term=NCT02434965&rank=1. Accessed 30 Nov 2015.
4. Carroll EJ, Sekul E, Bollag R, Ameri A, Neunert C, Johnson T et al. Safety and effectiveness of cord blood stem cell infusion for the treatment of cerebral palsy in children. 2010–2016. https://clinicaltrials.gov/ct2/show/NCT01072370?term=NCT01072370&rank=1. Accessed 30 Nov 2015.
5. Cotten MC, Fisher AK, Kurtzberg J, Song A, Goldstein R, Goldberg R et al. Cord blood for neonatal hypoxic-ischemic encephalopathy. 2008–2015. https://clinicaltrials.gov/ct2/show/NCT00593242?term=NCT00593242&rank=1. Accessed 30 Nov 2015.
6. Cox SC. Safety and effectiveness of banked cord blood or bone morrow stem cells in children with cerebral palsy (CP). (ACT for CP). 2013–2017. https://clinicaltrials.gov/ct2/show/NCT01988584?term=NCT01988584&rank=1. Accessed 30 Nov 2015.
7. Kim M. Allogeneic umbilical cord blood therapy for stroke. 2013–2015. https://clinicaltrials.gov/ct2/show/NCT01884155?term=NCT01884155&rank=1. Accessed 30 Nov 2015.
8. Kim M, Kang M, Kim S, Jang S, Min K, Lee J, et al. Allogeneic umbilical cord blood therapy in children with CP. 2013–2015. https://clinicaltrials.gov/ct2/show/NCT02025972?term=NCT02025972&rank=1. Accessed 30 Nov 2015.
9. Kim M, Kang M, Kim S, Jang S, Min K, Yoo S. Umbilical cord blood therapy for global developmental delay. 2012–2014. https://clinicaltrials.gov/ct2/show/NCT01769716?term=NCT01769716&rank=1. Accessed 30 Nov 2015.
10. Kim M, Kang M, Kim S, Jang S, Min K, Yoo S. UCB therapy in acquired brain injury. 2012–2014. https://clinicaltrials.gov/ct2/show/NCT01885663?term=UCB+Therapy+in+Acquired+Brain+Injury.&rank=1. Accessed 30 Nov 2015.
11. Kurtzberg J. A randomized study of autologous umbilical cord blood reinfusion in children with cerebral palsy. 2010–2016. https://clinicaltrials.gov/ct2/show/NCT01147653?term=NCT01147653&rank=1. Accessed 30 Nov 2015.
12. Kurtzberg J, Sun J. Assessment of the safety of allogeneic umbilical cord blood infusions in children with cerebral palsy. 2015–2018. https://clinicaltrials.gov/ct2/show/NCT02599207?term=NCT02599207&rank=1. Accessed 30 Nov 2015.
13. Lee J, Rajadurai S, Yeo LC. Autologous cord blood cells for brain injury in term newborns. 2011–2015. https://clinicaltrials.gov/ct2/show/NCT01649648?term=NCT01649648&rank=1. Accessed 30 Nov 2015.
14. Shintaku H. Autologous cord blood cell therapy for neonatal encephalopathy. 2014–2018. https://clinicaltrials.gov/ct2/show/NCT02256618?term=NCT02256618&rank=1. Accessed 30 Nov 2015.
15. Yin Z. Neuroprotective effect of autologous cord blood combined with therapeutic hypothermia following neonatal encephalopathy. 2015–2018. https://clinicaltrials.gov/ct2/show/NCT02605018?term=NCT02605018&rank=1. Accessed 30 Nov 2015.
16. Zhou W. Neuroprotective effect of autologous cord blood combined with therapeutic hypothermia following neonatal encephalopathy. 2015–2018. https://clinicaltrials.gov/ct2/show/NCT02551003?term=NCT02551003&rank=1. Accessed 30 Nov 2015.
17. Chen G, Wang Y, Xu Z, Fang F, Xu R, Hu X, et al. Neural stem cell-like cells derived from autologous bone mesenchymal stem cells for the treatment of patients with cerebral palsy. J Transl Med. 2013;11:21. https://doi.org/10.1186/1479-5876-11-21.
18. Cotten CM, Murtha AP, Goldberg RN, Grotegut CA, Smith PB, Goldstein RF, et al. Feasibility of autologous cord blood cells for infants with hypoxic-ischemic encephalopathy. J Pediatr. 2014;164(5):973–979.e1. https://doi.org/10.1016/j.jpeds.2013.11.036.
19. Kang M, Min K, Jang J, Kim SC, Kang MS, Jang SJ, et al. Involvement of immune responses in the efficacy of cord blood cell therapy for cerebral palsy. Stem Cells Dev. 2015;24(19):2259–68. https://doi.org/10.1089/scd.2015.0074.
20. Luan Z, Liu W, Qu S, Du K, He S, Wang Z, et al. Effects of neural progenitor cell transplantation in children with severe cerebral palsy. Cell Transplant. 2012;21(Suppl 1):S91–8. https://doi.org/10.3727/096368912X633806.

21. Luan Z, Qu S, Du K, Liu W, Yang Y, Wang Z, et al. Neural stem/progenitor cell transplantation for cortical visual impairment in neonatal brain injured patients. Cell Transplant. 2013;22(Suppl 1):S101–12. https://doi.org/10.3727/096368913X672163.
22. Hassan MA, Gabr H, Fathi S, Ramzy GM, El-Hassany AH, Abd El-Ghaffar NA. Stem cell transplantation in Egyptian patients with cerebral palsy. Egypt J Neuro Psychiat Neurosurg. 2012;49(2):117–22.
23. Mancias-Guerra C, Marroquin-Escamilla AR, Gonzalez-Llano O, Villarreal-Martinez L, Jaime-Perez JC, Garcia-Rodriguez F, et al. Safety and tolerability of intrathecal delivery of autologous bone marrow nucleated cells in children with cerebral palsy: an open-label phase I trial. Cytotherapy. 2014;16(6):810–20. https://doi.org/10.1016/j.jcyt.2014.01.008.
24. Min K, Song J, Kang JY, Ko J, Ryu JS, Kang MS, et al. Umbilical cord blood therapy potentiated with erythropoietin for children with cerebral palsy: a double-blind, randomized, placebo-controlled trial. Stem Cells. 2013;31(3):581–91. https://doi.org/10.1002/stem.1304.
25. Wang X, Cheng H, Hua R, Yang J, Dai G, Zhang Z, et al. Effects of bone marrow mesenchymal stromal cells on gross motor function measure scores of children with cerebral palsy: a preliminary clinical study. Cytotherapy. 2013;15(12):1549–62. https://doi.org/10.1016/j.jcyt.2013.06.001.
26. Pimentel-Coelho PM, Magalhaes ES, Lopes LM, deAzevedo LC, Santiago MF, Mendez-Otero R. Human cord blood transplantation in a neonatal rat model of hypoxic-ischemic brain damage: functional outcome related to neuroprotection in the striatum. Stem Cells Dev. 2010;19(3):351–8. https://doi.org/10.1089/scd.2009.0049.
27. Xia G, Hong X, Chen X, Lan F, Zhang G, Liao L. Intracerebral transplantation of mesenchymal stem cells derived from human umbilical cord blood alleviates hypoxic ischemic brain injury in rat neonates. J Perinat Med. 2010;38(2):215–21. https://doi.org/10.1515/JPM.2010.021.
28. Meier C, Middelanis J, Wasielewski B, Neuhoff S, Roth-Haerer A, Gantert M, et al. Spastic paresis after perinatal brain damage in rats is reduced by human cord blood mononuclear cells. Pediatr Res. 2006;59(2):244–9. https://doi.org/10.1203/01.pdr.0000197309.08852.f5.
29. MHLW. Ministry of Health, Labour and Welfare. http://www.mhlw.go.jp/english/. Accessed 11 Nov 2015.
30. PMDA. Pharmaceutical and Medical Devices Agency. http://www.pmda.go.jp/english/index.html. Accessed 11 Nov 2015.
31. FDA. U.S. Food and Drug Administration. http://www.fda.gov/default.htm. Accessed 11 Nov 2015.
32. EMA. European Medicines Agency. http://www.ema.europa.eu/ema/. Accessed 11 Nov 2015.
33. ICH. The international council for harmonisation of technical requirements for pharmaceuticals for human use. http://www.ich.org/home.html. Accessed 11 Nov 2015.

Chapter 14
A New Prospective Cell Therapy for Neonatal Brain Injury

Tokiko Nagamura-Inoue

Abstract Cerebral palsy is a lifelong neurological disorder, mainly caused by hypoxic-ischemic encephalopathy, hemorrhage, and periventricular leukomalacia occurring at delivery or perinatally. To prevent or reduce the neurogenic disabilities in cerebral palsy, therapies using hypothermia, autologous cord blood infusion, and recently, mesenchymal stromal cells (MSCs) have been applied. MSCs can be obtained from fetal appendages such as cord blood, umbilical cord, amnion, and placenta. In this chapter, the expected feasibility of such cell therapies for cerebral palsy is discussed.

Keywords Mesenchymal stromal cells · Umbilical cord · Perinatal brain injury Neurogenic differentiation

14.1 Cell Therapy Principles: Past and Present

Cerebral palsy (CP) is a lifelong neurogenic disorder affecting motor development, and its main causes are periventricular leukomalacia (PVL), hypoxic-ischemic encephalopathy (HIE) at delivery, and intraventricular hemorrhage (IVH) followed by posthemorrhagic hydrocephalus (PHH). The mechanism of development into CP from PVL, HIE, and IVH varies and is complicated. The inflammatory cytokine storm and degeneration of neurons in the brain occur in the acute phase, as described in Chaps. 3–5 of this book. At present, once neurological disabilities are established, resolving them is difficult.

Currently, hypothermia therapy is the only standard procedure to prevent progression to CP. Kurtzberg et al. reported that autologous cord blood (CB) infusion could improve motor function even in infants, and this finding provided enormous

T. Nagamura-Inoue, M.D., Ph.D.
Department of Cell Processing and Transfusion, Research Hospital,
The Institute of Medical Science, The University of Tokyo, Tokyo, Japan
e-mail: tokikoni@ims.u-tokyo.ac.jp

© Springer Nature Singapore Pte Ltd. 2018

H. Shintaku et al. (eds.), *Cell Therapy for Perinatal Brain Injury*,
https://doi.org/10.1007/978-981-10-1412-3_14

hope in the field of perinatal and neonatal medicine. Transplanting CB CD34-positive cells [1] or CD133-positive stem cells [2] in a mouse model of cerebral injuries demonstrated the presence of human cells differentiating in the mouse brain, as well as keeping white matter of the mouse brain.

Some researchers demonstrated that mesenchymal stromal cells (MSCs) can be obtained from cultured CB cells, but few MSCs are found in primary CB cells. Very small embryonic stem-like (VSEL) cells in CB are characterized by pluripotency, as reported by Ratajack et al. [3], although the published findings could not be replicated by other researchers because of the very small sample size and limited amount of CB. At present, CD34/CD133-positive cells in CB may play a critical role in regenerative medicine for CP in animal models. Because of the correlation of CD34-positive cells and CB volume, the amount of autologous CB collected at birth is an important factor for the success of improving CP. On the other hand, CB includes not only hematopoietic stem cells but also regulatory innate immune cells in the specila manner in the uterus, including macrophages, regulatory T cells, B cells, NK cells [4], and NKT cells [5, 6]. Immediately after birth, a baby's immune system is activated and initiated to respond to the external environment. The perinatal phase is a very delicate stage for a newborn, and it remained unknown whether the immune cells in the infused CB play an important role to regulate the cytokine storm in the acute phase of cerebral damage *in vivo*.

At present, minimally manipulated autologous CB therapy for CP is a simple and feasible approach in the early phase of neurological injuries, although CB processing requires trained physicians and technicians in each hospital, if they process CB in-house. However, CB infusion therapy is beset by various limitations posed by CB collection, such as technique, timing, size of placenta, and immaturity of the baby. All these factors may influence the volume of CB collected.

14.2 New Cell Therapy Source for Cerebral Palsy

Recently, MSCs have demonstrated promising functions not only for multipotent ability but also for anti-inflammatory ability and acceleration of tissue repair. Numerous papers have reported that MSCs have clinical relevance for various diseases, including severe acute graft-versus-host disease (GVHD) after hematopoietic stem cell transplantation (HSCT), Crohn's disease, cerebral infarction, spinal dissection, and certain collagen diseases. MSCs can be harvested from various tissues, such as bone marrow (BM) [7], CB [8], adipose tissue [9], placenta [10], and umbilical cord (UC) [11]. UC and other fetal appendages may also be collected easily at birth even after CB collection, although maintaining their post-collection safety and quality until autologous use may be time-consuming and costly. BM-derived MSCs are successfully being applied for clinical use in adult patients. In particular, autologous BM-MSCs used for cerebral infarctions were found to improve motor function [12]. The next MSC source for HSCT is derived from allogeneic donors. In the treatment of severe acute GVHD, third party donor-derived BM-MSCs were reported to have the same effect on severe acute GVHD as HSCT donor-derived MSCs. The fact that third party-derived MSCs have the equivalent immunosuppressive potential has extended the possibility to use off-the-shelf MSCs derived from fetal appendages. Moreover, MSCs do not express co-stimulatory surface antigens that activate T cells, such as CD40, CD80, or CD86 [13]. Thus, MSCs escape activated T cells and exert immunomodulatory effects. The authors reported that allogeneic UC-MSCs have immunosuppressive effects and a potential to differentiate into neurogenic progenitors, accompanied with the ability to migrate to injured cells [14]. Several researchers reported the usefulness of UC-MSCs using the animal models of neonatal brain injuries, such as IVH [15], PVL, and cerebral infarction and some of them progressed into clinical trials [16]. The authors are now preparing off-the-shelf UC-MSCs banking, samples of which are ready-to-use upon request. Allogeneic UC-MSCs can be expanded, and large amounts of UC-MSCs are cryopreserved in a commercial base [15, 16], while autologous ones are processed by in-house processing. UCs may also be collected and transferred to the processing center. The cost and benefit should be calculated based on scientific proof. Details of the possibility to use UC-MSCs for CP as regenerative field are discussed in Chap. 6.

The mechanism of the immunosuppressive effect by MSCs has been explored [17–20]. At the onset of PVL, HIE, and IVH followed by PHH, a series of inflammatory cytokines and superoxides may activate MSCs as immune-regulators. MSCs may suppress not only T cells but also monocytes, NK cells [21], and B cells via different mechanisms. The immunomodulation may be linked to soluble factors such as indoleamine 2,3-dioxygenase (IDO) [22], prostaglandin E2, transforming growth factor-β1, galectin-1, HLA-G5 [23], hepatocyte growth factor, and interleukin-10 released from MSCs [24]. In some studies, exosomes and soluble factors of conditioned culture media of MSCs are also effective not only for immunosuppression but also for differentiation of MSCs into neurogenic progenitors. Nevertheless, the specific mechanisms of immune modulation by UC-MSCs remain undefined.

14.3 Prospective Study of Cell Therapy for CP

Figure 14.1 shows an example of prospective cell therapy for CP or pre-CP status in the near future. The causes of CP are divided into two groups by period of onset. One occurs in the perinatal period, including placenta previa, UC prolapse, placental ablation, UC loop, and maternal shock. The other occurs in the postpartum period, such as cerebral hemorrhage, PVL, subgaleal hematoma, and cerebral infarction. If the affected babies are delivered at full term without the complication of IVH, autologous CB collection can be done. Such babies are also applicable for hypothermia therapy. However, premature babies (delivery before 36 gestational weeks) or those with IVH complication are excluded from autologous CB collection and infusion. Moreover, even if CB is collected, the amount is too small to manipulate and infuse and is therefore excluded for clinical studies. These cases might be rescued by UC collection, although the use of autologous UC-MSCs remains to be evaluated. The quality and safety of UCs derived from the patients needs to be checked, including genetic abnormalities during the culture of UC-MSCs. Alternatively, allogeneic ready-to-use UC-MSCs, which are collected from healthy donors with normal delivery, are available. The infusion of CB and

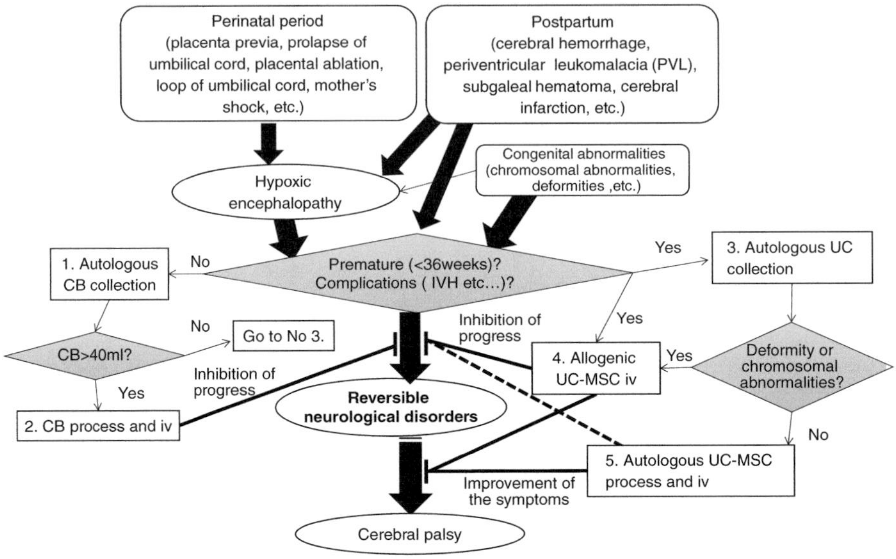

Fig. 14.1 Flowchart of the prospective cell therapy for cerebral palsy

allogeneic UC-MSCs is expected to prevent the development to CP, while autologous UC-MSCs might improve the symptoms of established CP. Cell therapies for CP prevention and treatment have just begun and should continue to be explored, particularly in terms of autologous or allogeneic donor origin, timing of infusion, reflecting the pathogenesis, and mechanism of action.

14.4 Conclusion

Minimally manipulated CB therapies for cell therapies are still advancing. UC-MSC therapy is a recently introduced new approach that is expected to help prevent or improve CP progression. These cell therapies for CP should be based on the proof of concept supported by fundamental scientific experiments related to the pathogenesis of the onset of CP.

References

1. Tsuji M, Taguchi A, Ohshima M, Kasahara Y, Sato Y, Tsuda H, et al. Effects of intravenous administration of umbilical cord blood CD34(+) cells in a mouse model of neonatal stroke. Neuroscience. 2014;263:148–58. Epub 2014/01/22.
2. Jang YK, Park JJ, Lee MC, Yoon BH, Yang YS, Yang SE, et al. Retinoic acid-mediated induction of neurons and glial cells from human umbilical cord-derived hematopoietic stem cells. J Neurosci Res. 2004;75(4):573–84. Epub 2004/01/27.

3. Ratajczak MZ, Zuba-Surma EK, Shin DM, Ratajczak J, Kucia M. Very small embryonic-like (VSEL) stem cells in adult organs and their potential role in rejuvenation of tissues and longevity. Exp Gerontol. 2008;43(11):1009–17. Epub 2008/07/08.
4. Nagamura-Inoue T, Mori Y, Yizhou Z, Watanabe N, Takahashi TA. Differential expansion of umbilical cord blood mononuclear cell-derived natural killer cells dependent on the dose of interleukin-15 with Flt3L. Exp Hematol. 2004;32(2):202–9. Epub 2004/04/23.
5. Hikaru Okada, Tokiko Nagamura-Inoue, Yuka Mori, Tsuneo A. Takahashi, Expansion of Vα 24+Vβ 11 NKT cells from cord blood mononuclear cells using IL-15, IL-7 and Flt3-L depends on monocytes. European Journal of Immunology. 2006;36(1):236–44.
6. Cany J, Dolstra H, Shah N. Umbilical cord blood-derived cellular products for cancer immunotherapy. Cytotherapy. 2015;17(6):739–48. Epub 2015/03/22.
7. Gnecchi M, Melo LG. Bone marrow-derived mesenchymal stem cells: isolation, expansion, characterization, viral transduction, and production of conditioned medium. Methods Mol Biol. 2009;482:281–94. Epub 2008/12/18.
8. Bieback K, Kluter H. Mesenchymal stromal cells from umbilical cord blood. Curr Stem Cell Res Ther. 2007;2(4):310–23.
9. Gruber HE, Deepe R, Hoelscher GL, Ingram JA, Norton HJ, Scannell B, et al. Human adipose-derived mesenchymal stem cells: direction to a phenotype sharing similarities with the disc, gene expression profiling, and coculture with human annulus cells. Tissue Eng A. 2010;16(9):2843–60. Epub 2010/04/23.
10. In't Anker PS, Scherjon SA, Kleijburg-van der Keur C, de Groot-Swings GM, Claas FH, Fibbe WE, et al. Isolation of mesenchymal stem cells of fetal or maternal origin from human placenta. Stem Cells. 2004;22(7):1338–45.
11. Romanov YA, Svintsitskaya VA, Smirnov VN. Searching for alternative sources of postnatal human mesenchymal stem cells: candidate MSC-like cells from umbilical cord. Stem Cells. 2003;21(1):105–10.
12. Ukai R, Honmou O, Harada K, Houkin K, Hamada H, Kocsis JD. Mesenchymal stem cells derived from peripheral blood protects against ischemia. J Neurotrauma. 2007;24(3):508–20.
13. Weiss ML, Anderson C, Medicetty S, Seshareddy KB, Weiss RJ, VanderWerff I, et al. Immune properties of human umbilical cord Wharton's jelly-derived cells. Stem Cells. 2008;26(11):2865–74. Epub 2008/08/16.
14. Takeo Mukai, Tokiko Nagamura-Inoue, Takahisa Shimazu, Yuka Mori, Atsuko Takahashi, Hajime Tsunoda, Satoru Yamaguchi, Arinobu Tojo, Neurosphere formation enhances the neurogenic differentiation potential and migratory ability of umbilical cord-mesenchymal stromal cells. Cytotherapy. 2016;18(2):229–41.
15. Mukai T, Mori Y, Shimazu T, Takahashi A, Tsunoda H, Yamaguchi S, et al. Intravenous injection of umbilical cord-derived mesenchymal stromal cells attenuates reactive gliosis and hypomyelination in a neonatal intraventricular hemorrhage model. Neuroscience. 2017;355:175–87. Epub 2017/05/16.
16. Nagamura-Inoue T, Mukai T. Umbilical Cord is a Rich Source of Mesenchymal Stromal Cells for Cell Therapy. Current stem cell research & therapy. 2016;11(8):634–42. Epub 2015/10/27.
17. English K, Barry FP, Mahon BP. Murine mesenchymal stem cells suppress dendritic cell migration, maturation and antigen presentation. Immunol Lett. 2008;115(1):50–8. Epub 2007/11/21.
18. Spaggiari GM, Capobianco A, Abdelrazik H, Becchetti F, Mingari MC, Moretta L. Mesenchymal stem cells inhibit natural killer-cell proliferation, cytotoxicity, and cytokine production: role of indoleamine 2,3-dioxygenase and prostaglandin E2. Blood. 2008;111(3):1327–33. Epub 2007/10/24.
19. Asari S, Itakura S, Ferreri K, Liu CP, Kuroda Y, Kandeel F, et al. Mesenchymal stem cells suppress B-cell terminal differentiation. Exp Hematol. 2009;37(5):604–15. Epub 2009/04/21.
20. Magatti M, De Munari S, Vertua E, Gibelli L, Wengler GS, Parolini O. Human amnion mesenchyme harbors cells with allogeneic T-cell suppression and stimulation capabilities. Stem Cells. 2008;26(1):182–92. Epub 2007/09/29.
21. Noone C, Kihm A, English K, O'Dea S, Mahon BP. IFN-gamma stimulated human umbilical-tissue-derived cells potently suppress NK activation and resist NK-mediated cytotoxicity in vitro. Stem Cells Dev. 2013;22(22):3003–14. Epub 2013/06/26.

22. He H, Nagamura-Inoue T, Takahashi A, Mori Y, Yamamoto Y, Shimazu T, et al. Immunosuppressive properties of Wharton's jelly-derived mesenchymal stromal cells in vitro. Int J Hematol. 2015;102(3):368–78. Epub 2015/08/01.
23. Seshareddy K, Troyer D, Weiss ML. Method to isolate mesenchymal-like cells from Wharton's Jelly of umbilical cord. Methods Cell Biol. 2008;86:101–19. Epub 2008/04/30.
24. Zhou C, Yang B, Tian Y, Jiao H, Zheng W, Wang J, et al. Immunomodulatory effect of human umbilical cord Wharton's jelly-derived mesenchymal stem cells on lymphocytes. Cell Immunol. 2011;272(1):33–8. Epub 2011/10/19.

MIX
Papier aus verantwortungsvollen Quellen
Paper from responsible sources
FSC® C105338

If you have any concerns about our products,
you can contact us on
ProductSafety@springernature.com

In case Publisher is established outside the EU,
the EU authorized representative is:
Springer Nature Customer Service Center GmbH
Europaplatz 3, 69115 Heidelberg, Germany

Printed by Libri Plureos GmbH
in Hamburg, Germany